FUNDAMENTALS OF DISEASE AND INSECT CONTROL

FUNDAMENTALS OF DISEASE AND INSECT CONTROL

Editor
Gove Hambidge

BIOTECH
2025
BIOTECH BOOKS

ISBN 978-81-7622-083-5

Published by: **BIOTECH BOOKS®**
4762-63/23, Ansari Road, Darya Ganj,
New Delhi - 110 002
Phone: 09899295259, 011-43003222
E-mail: biotechbooks@yahoo.co.in
Website: www.biotechbooks.in

Typeset at: **Classic Computer Services**
Delhi - 110 035

PRINTED IN INDIA

CONTENTS

INTRODUCTION

Losses Caused by Animal Diseases And Parasites

J.R. Mohler, Wight, MacKellar, and Bishopp give a broad picture of the nature as well as the extent of the losses caused by livestock diseases and internal and external parasites in this country. Only a few selected cases can actually be covered, and there is little doubt that the total figure for losses quoted at the end of the article ($418,000,000 a year) is an underestimate rather than an overestimate.

There are four main things that can be done to keep such losses within reasonable bounds in the crowded livestock population of today: (1) Aggressive research can discover how to combat livestock enemies. (2) Vigilant regulation can prevent the spread of certain diseases and safeguard the public's food supply. (3) Extensive campaigns of eradication can reduce especially dangerous diseases to a minimum. (4) Losses could be enormously reduced if all farmers and others directly concerned with the livestock industry would adopt sound practices in their everyday operations. For example, it has been estimated that losses due to preventable injuries in the shipping of livestock amount to 11.5 million dollars a year. Great numbers of animals are unnecessarily lost every year, or fail to produce what they should, because management practices that would prevent ordinary diseases and parasites from getting a foothold are not followed on the farm.

A few diseases are considered separately in the article. The record in the case of cattle tuberculosis is excellent; the campaign of testing and slaughter has brought this disease to a very low point in less than 25 years. There is considerable avian tuberculosis in poultry, however, and most of the tuberculosis in swine is of the avian type, spread by poultry. The outlook for successfully combating brucellosis of cattle (Bang's disease) is good; this campaign was begun in 1934, and results are very promising. In the case of Johne's disease, which is incurable, a diagnostic skin test has been developed that makes it possible to eliminate diseased animals. Cattle tick fever has been reduced to negligible proportions by an extensive eradication campaign. Hog cholera is still the most destructive disease of swine, but present immunization methods prevent the devastating periodic outbreaks of the past.

Much of the loss from internal parasites is indirect, taking the form of stunted growth, ill health, reduced production, and condemned meat products; but conservative estimates indicate that these parasites rob the country of at least 125 million dollars a year. It has been amply proved both in experimental work and in farm practice that these losses can be sharply reduced by effective medication and the use of sound control measures, including good sanitation especially.

In the case of insects, much of the loss is also indirect, and part of it is due to the sheer tormenting of the animals by the more vicious insect enemies. The grubs or maggots of certain insects are serious internal parasites; lice and mites in heavy infestations do an immense amount of damage; and one of the worst aspects of the insect menace is that several dangerous diseases of animals and human beings are spread by these creatures. Not all insects can be successfully combated at present, but many can be, and the damage done by others can at least be reduced.

Causes of Diseases

"Disease," says Schoening, who writes the first part of this article, dealing with bacteria and viruses, "may be defined as any abnormal condition of the tissues of the body." Such an abnormal condition may be due to injuries (wounds, contusions), bacteria, viruses, internal and external parasites, chemicals, poisons of various kinds, faulty nutrition, and inherited abnormalities. When cells are damaged by a disease agent, the body hastens to repair the injury, and the repair process sets up an inflammation, indicated in medical language by the ending "itis". Hence the names of many diseases end in itis–for example, appendicitis, an inflammation of the appendix.

Bacteria are minute living things visible only under a microscope. They are distinguished and classified by such differences as those in size, shape, the conditions under which they can grow, the kind of food they can utilize, and their effects on experimental animals. They exist everywhere in nature, and many of them perform necessary or useful functions, while others produce disease. Some can move around on their own power, others cannot. Some can go into a resting, or spore, stage during which they are especially resistant to destruction. Some–diphtheria germs, for instance–produce powerful poisons called soluble toxins. Some produce abscesses or other local inflammations that under the right conditions can set up a general poisoning of the system, or septicemia.

Viruses are too small to be seen under a microscope, and they pass through a filter fine enough to hold back bacteria. Only in recent years has it been possible to propagate some viruses artificially, by the use of living tissues; and these studies have revealed many facts and led to the development of certain immunization methods. More than 35 virus diseases of animals are now known. Some viruses attack nerve tissue primarily, as in rabies and encephalomyelitis; others, skin and membrane tissues, as in foot-and-mouth disease; and still others, several or all kinds of tissue. After a virus has weakened the body's; defences, bacteria that may not ordinarily be very harmful will often become secondary invaders, with serious results, as in hog cholera complications.

Bacteria and viruses invade the body in various ways, mainly through the respiratory, digestive, and genital tracts and the skin. They are transmitted from animal to animal by biting insects, by the blood, excretions, and secretions of infected animals which contaminate the surroundings, and by carriers–that is, animals that harbour an infective agent without apparently getting the disease themselves or continue to harbour the agent after recovering, as in foot-and-mouth disease.

Whether an infective agent actually causes a disease in any given case depends on the resistance of the host and the virulence of the agent. Some disease organisms (anthrax bacteria in the spore stage, for instance) are very resistant to destruction and can live for a long time outside an animal's body.

Malaria, African sleeping sickness, and amoebic dysentery are examples of diseases of human beings caused by internal parasites. There is no hard-and-fast line, says Schwartz, who writes the section on parasites, between such diseases and those produced by bacteria and viruses, though the parasitic diseases are likely to develop more slowly and less noticeably. Perhaps all animals harbour some parasites, but comparatively few of the many species are of major importance to animal and human health. A peculiarity of many internal parasites is that they cannot go through their entire life cycle in a single kind of animal; part of their development must take place in a different kind of animal, called an intermediate host, and this often complicates the problem of control. The intermediate host takes in the eggs or larvae of the parasite; then the final host takes in the intermediate host or some infected part of it, or acquires the parasites by being bitten by infective intermediate hosts such as ticks and mosquitoes.

There are two broad groups of internal parasites–the protozoa (minute one-celled animals) and the helminths, or worms.

Protozoa multiply rapidly in the animal body, either by division or by a process resembling sexual reproduction, and often cause severe diseases. Some protozoa have only one host, and infection takes place through food or water contaminated by droppings–as in the case of amoebic dysentery, blackhead, and coccidiosis, the last one often a serious disease of poultry, cattle, and sheep–or through some other direct means. In other cases, the protozoa are transmitted only through agents known as vectors–the cattle tick fever organism through ticks, for instance.

The worm parasites range in length, as adults, from a small fraction of an inch to several feet. They are often equipped with spines, hooks, teeth, or suckers to attach themselves, and they can move around in the host's body. Helminths reproduce sexually by means of eggs, and in most cases the eggs or young larvae must leave the host's body and go through one or more stages of development in the open or in intermediate hosts. Infection takes place through the swallowing of contaminated feed or water, penetration of larvae through the skin, the swallowing of intermediate hosts, or the bites of insects. Practically all the tissues and organs of the body are subject to attack by various kinds of worms, including all parts of the digestive tract and abdominal cavity, the skin and muscles, the liver, pancreas, spleen, and kidneys, the heart, lungs, brain, eyes. Severe hemorrhages, anemia, emaciation, and death are common results of heavy infections by some worm parasites.

Of the three main groups of worms, (1) the flukes require snails as intermediate hosts (flukes that attack the liver of animals are the only ones of importance in this country); (2) the tapeworms occur as adults in the intestine and as bladder worms (immature forms) in the muscles, abdominal cavity, liver, lungs, brain, eyes, and elsewhere, and they require intermediate hosts, which include mites, lice, fleas, beetles, and higher animals; and (3) the roundworms, or nematodes, occur in practically all parts of the body, often wander extensively, and are among the most injurious of parasites, causing such serious maladies as trichinosis and hookworm disease. Some nematodes require intermediate hosts, and some do not.

Modern discoveries concerning nutritional diseases have been as dramatic and important as the earlier discoveries that established infections as causes of disease, Madsen points out, and they have made it possible to guard against many dangers not understood in the past. Since Madsen takes up the nutritional diseases of livestock at length elsewhere in this volume, his discussion here is very brief and general.

Plant poisoning is also discussed at some length elsewhere in the volume. Here Couch points out certain general facts, such as: Some parts of a plant are likely to be more poisonous than other parts, and the poison may affect certain species of animals more than others. There is a great deal of variation in the symptoms and the injuries caused by poisonous plants because of the many different toxic substances involved, and sometimes these symptoms can easily be mistaken for those of other diseases. Moreover, plants that are not poisonous in themselves sometimes take up toxic substances from the soil–as in the case of selenium particularly–in sufficient quantities to be damaging or deadly to livestock.

Protective Mechanisms Against Disease

The body is equipped by nature to fight against disease. Among its chief defences are certain large cells called phagocytes, which can devour invading disease organisms. Under the stimulus of a particular invading organism, the phagocytes can also produce antibodies capable of destroying it or neutralizing its poisons (toxins). Through many years of research, medical science has learned how to immunize animals and human beings against certain diseases by either stimulating this process, producing what is called active immunity, or supplementing it, producing what is called passive immunity.

In a sense, active immunity is induced by giving the animal a mild or modified case of the disease. Some of the virus, the germs, or the toxins, usually in a weakened form, are injected into the animal. This sets its defence mechanism to work producing antibodies. Then, if the animal should be attacked by the disease at some time in the future, the antibodies are already there to fight the invasion; in other words, the animal is immune. It usually takes a week or two to produce active immunity, but it lasts a long time because the animal keeps on manufacturing antibodies.

In case a disease threatens in the immediate future or has already attacked, it may be desirable to produce passive immunity. This is done by taking immune bodies out of another animal, usually in its blood serum, and injecting them into the animal to be protected. Such borrowed immunity acts at once (it may also have a curative effect), but it does not last long because the borrowed immune bodies gradually disappear; they are not continuously produced in the animal's own body.

Sometimes both active and passive immunity are produced at the same time by injecting the disease organism or toxin plus immune bodies from another animal. This is the method called simultaneous vaccination.

Disease organisms and toxins are treated in various ways, described by Eichhorn, to make them relatively harmless to the animal getting the injection or injections. The whole process is usually extremely delicate and exact. As the author points out, however, much more is involved in effective immunization than merely using these biological products. Everything possible should be done to build up the animal's general health and vigour and to eliminate the sources of infection; and exactly the right techniques must be used in preparing, handling, and administering the biological products themselves.

Certain biological products, called diagnostic agents, have been developed for detecting the presence of a disease, even when it shows no outward signs. Two of these tests, the complement-fixation test and the agglutination test, are described by Eichhorn.

In the case of internal parasites, Sarles points out, the existence of any protective mechanism or immunity was considered to be improbable until a few years ago. Now it is known that immunity both natural and acquired, against parasites does exist and that it is basically similar to immunity against virus and bacterial infections. Antibodies are evidently of primary importance in acquired immunity to parasites–so much so that immune serum can be used to transfer immunity to susceptible animals. Adequate methods of artificial immunization against parasites have not been developed, however, and for practical purposes it is necessary to depend on the recognized means of prevention and treatment of parasitism.

There can be no doubt, Ellis indicates, that good nutrition is essential if the animal body is to combat and counteract disease-producing organisms; but evidence that any specific nutritive factor has a direct relationship to the mechanism of immunity, in the medical sense, is still inconclusive. Vitamin A may contribute to resistance by keeping the tissues of the lining membranes from breaking down, but artificial injections of disease organisms tend to prove that the vitamin does more than this. In the case of vitamin B_1, possibly the lowered body temperature and the lack of appetite associated with a deficiency may decrease the ability of the body to produce phagocytes, or devouring cells. Other dietary factors discussed by Ellis in their relationship to certain infectious diseases include vitamin D, nicotinic acid, protein, and calcium.

The Endocrine Glands in Health and Disease

The hormones secreted by the endocrine glands have such extraordinary effects in the animal body that to the layman they sometimes seem almost magical. As Frank points out, much research in this field is now under way, and it holds great promise for the future. He briefly describes the chief functions of the nine glands.

The pituitary gland, at the base of the brain, has two parts, or lobes. The anterior, or upper, lobe may well be called the master gland of the body. It secretes at least eleven complex hormones. Two of these, the gonadotropic hormones, act directly on the gonads (ovaries of the female and testicles of the male), and extracts are used medically (one is used in a test for pregnancy after breeding). A third hormone (the mammogenic) stimulates the development of the mammary glands of the breasts or udder; a fourth (the lactogenic) stimulates the production of milk; a fifth directly influences growth, an excess producing giants and a deficiency dwarfs; a sixth apparently has an indirect influence on calcium metabolism; a seventh controls a very vital part of the adrenal glands; an eighth influences carbohydrate metabolism; possibly a ninth influences fat and protein digestion; a tenth governs the activity of the thyroid gland; and an eleventh influences the secretion of insulin by the pancreas.

The posterior (lower) lobe of the pituitary secretes pituitrin, which stimulates the muscles of the uterus at parturition, the small blood vessels, the intestines, and, in females, the mammary glands. Pituitrin is valuable medically.

The male gonads secrete the male sex hormone, testosterone, which, among other functions, is responsible for the development of secondary sex characters. It has been made synthetically and is used in medical practice. The female gonads secrete the two female sex hormones, estrogen and progestin. The former (also produced synthetically and used in medical practice) acts directly on the female sex organs and is concerned in the sex cycle, including estrus, or heat. Progestin acts with estrogen to stimulate the production of the mammogenic hormone by the pituitary.

Four other glands are very important. The parathyroids, in the neck, produce a hormone that is responsible for maintaining the balance between calcium and phosphorus in the body. The adrenal glands (one in front of each kidney) have (1) an inner (medullary) part secreting adrenin, which acts like pituitrin and is used medically as a heart stimulant and to check hemorrhages, and (2) an outer (cortical) part secreting cortin, without which an animal cannot stay alive. The thyroid gland, in the neck, secretes thyroxin, which controls the energy output of the body and needs iodine for its formation; a deficiency of thyroxin results in goiter, cretinism, and other abnormal conditions. The pancreas gland, near the stomach, secretes digestive juices and the hormone insulin, which is necessary for the proper utilization of sugar by the body.

Little is known about the functions of two other glands–the pineal, in the central part of the brain, and the thymus, which is well developed in young animals (the so-called sweetbread of calves) but degenerates at maturity.

The Relation of Genetics to Disease

Plant breeders have not only proved that disease resistance is inherited; many of their greatest triumphs have been due to the breeding of resistant varieties. Can the same thing be done with animals?

As proof that it can, McPhee cites Lambert's work with fowl typhoid. By injecting White Leghorns with fowl typhoid bacteria and using only the most resistant individuals for breeding, Lambert reduced the mortality from this disease by about 90 percent in the fifth generation. Similar, though not such extreme, results have been obtained in experiments with mouse typhoid and with pullorum disease of chickens. Recently, in California, pigs have been discovered that apparently transmit resistance to brucellosis of swine.

Theoretically, then, it should be just as possible to cut death losses from certain diseases in half by breeding as it is to double egg production by breeding. The question is whether it can be done on a practical basis. It is expensive to develop and maintain a resistant line; the animals must be deliberately inoculated to prove that they are resistant; and a single outcross to a susceptible animal means that the work has to be done all over again. But, says McPhee, the case for or against the practical use of inherited resistance has never been proved because in no single instance has an experiment been carried far enough to see whether it might have practical applications. He believes there is evidence that warrants optimism for the not too distant future.

Popularly, a vigourous animal is supposed to be resistant to disease, but McPhee cites experiments which show that the various elements making for vigour are inherited independently of disease resistance. Again theoretically, however, vigour and disease resistance might be twin goals in a breeding project.

It is well known that the virulence of a disease organism changes. Is this due to environment, or does the organism itself mutate and hybridize? We cannot find out much about it, says McPhee, until we first have animals of known genetic constitution on which to test the organism. Otherwise it is always possible that apparent changes in virulence may really be due to variations in the host animals.

At the end of his article, the author describes various abnormalities in cattle, horses, sheep, swine, and poultry, the mode of inheritance of which is known. Many of these abnormalities are lethal–that is, the animals in which they appear cannot survive–and most are recessives. When such a recessive shows up, the sire, the dam, and all their off-spring should be discarded for breeding purposes.

Artificial Insemination and Disease Control

Artificial insemination of dairy cows is now widely practiced in the United States. This method of breeding has been used also to some extent with other domestic animals and poultry. In the main, the object is to increase the usefulness of outstanding sires, but the technique is also helpful in controlling diseases spread by sexual contact. Among these, Frank and Phillips list granular vaginitis of cattle, abortion in cows caused by an organism called *Vibrio fetus*, trichomoniasis of cows, navel ill of foals, dourine of horses, possibly brucellosis of cattle and of swine, coital exanthema of horses, and vent gleet of poultry.

From the standpoint of disease control, the essentials are (1) the selection of males known to be free from disease, and (2) absolute cleanliness and the sterilization of all instruments used in the collection and transfer of seminal fluid. The latter precaution is extremely important because instruments used on an infected female might transfer the infection to another female even if the male were completely free from disease.

Disinfection and Disinfectants

The first step in preventing infection, says Tilley, is cleanliness; proper cleaning removes most germs, and with clean animals in clean surroundings there will usually be no need for disinfectants unless disease breaks out.

There is no such thing as a general disinfectant; different disinfectants are effective against different germs, and even then other conditions are important also. In general, in using a disinfectant, (1) do a thorough cleaning job first, leaving as little dirt as possible, (2) allow plenty of time for the disinfectant to act, (3) use it warm or hot if possible, (4) apply it liberally and thoroughly. A spray pump is best for large areas; a whitewash brush can be used for small ones.

Simple, inexpensive disinfectants can usually be used in place of more expensive preparations. Lime and lye are two of the cheapest.

Tilley goes into the practical details neccessary to use the following substances or methods, giving the chief limitations of each and indicating whether it will or will not kill certain especially resistant germs and spores of disease.

Heat

Dry heat, in an ordinary oven, and mois theat–boiling water or steam–are both effective when properly applied.

Sulfur Dioxide

Not classed as a good germicide.

Formaldehyde

May be used as a gas under certain conditions, or as a solution with a high disinfecting power.

Boric Acid

A cleansing agent with little power to kill germs.

Acetic Acid

More potent than boric acid. Full-strength vinegar will kill some of the less resistant disease germs.

Lime

Widely useful. Quicklime only should be used to prepare slaked lime, milk of lime, and whitewash.

Lye

Also very useful. May be mixed in whitewash. Is a caustic poison and should be used with caution.

Sodium Carbonate (washing soda, soda crystals, soda ash)

Chiefly a cleansing agent but has some disinfecting value.

Trisodium Phosphate (tribasic phosphate of soda)

About like sodium carbonate.

Sulfate of Copper (blue vitriol)

Effective against algae.

Chloride of Lime (bleaching powder)

A powerful disinfectant, but not very practical for various reasons, including its odour, which is readily absorbed by food products.

Hypochlorites

Often employed to sterilize dairy equipment but useless unless the equipment is thoroughly cleaned first.

Iodine (tincture of iodine)

The standard substance for skin disinfection and treatment of surface wounds.

Alcohol (70 percent)

Effective against the less resistant disease germs.

Carbolic Acid (phenol)

Has several disadvantages but can sometimes be used on a small scale.

Cresol

Better and more powerful than carbolic acid. Especially useful in a soap solution (compound solution of cresol or saponified cresol). Also occurs mixed with coal-tar oils and soap in coal-tar emulsion disinfectants.

Soaps

Valuable chiefly for cleanliness. Their germicidal power is limited.

How Research Aids in Diseases Control

The Chief of the Bureau of Animal Industry here discusses some of the problems of research in animal disease and tells how research works and what it accomplishes.

A typical problem: A good many years ago certain swine growers called for help. What, they asked, was causing half their young pigs to die and stunting many of the survivors? Investigation showed that the swine were infested with ascarids, or roundworms.

Close study of the life cycle of this parasite showed the conditions under which it could survive and spread–and those were exactly the conditions under which pigs were commonly farrowed and raised. On the basis of this study, a radical new system was worked out to prevent infestation–a sort of combination of maternity hospital and pasture parlor for swine. Farmers tried this system out for 6 years. It worked, eliminating 98 percent of the parasite infestations and filth-borne diseases. It is now widely used.

Mohler lists many fundamental discoveries and advances made by veterinary research, some of which apply to human as well as animal diseases. A few of them: Simultaneous injection of immune serum and virulent blood as a means of immunization; proof that certain diseases can be carried from one animal to another only by an intermediate insect host; discovery that hog cholera is caused by a virus, and development of methods of immunization; discovery of a remedy for hookworm in dogs that has been successfully used for millions of human beings; discovery of phenothiazine as an anthelmintic; development of a vaccine to combat encephalomyelitis (sleeping sickness) of horses–a disease that is also a menace to human beings. Research work is back of meat-inspection service, which protects the health of consumers; the improvements made in the handling of livestock and livestock products in interstate and foreign trade; and advancements in the standards of veterinary education and practice.

Research projects now being carried on under congressional authorization include studies in brucellosis of cattle, mastitis of cattle, tuberculosis, Johne's disease, nutritional deficiencies of cattle, bovine trichomoniasis of cattle, anaplasmosis of cattle, equine encephalomyelitis, rabies, swine erysipelas, swine influenza, periodic ophthalmia of horses, hog cholera, and many other diseases, including parasitic diseases in general and various diseases of poultry. Fundamental investigation of the mechanisms of infection and of methods of control for all kinds of diseases is also in progress. The Federal research work on disease subjects is done in various parts of the country, and much of it is in cooperation with the States.

Mohler shows that in the course of their work, research men sometimes risk health and even life in the service of science. The results of the work, most of which is directed toward the solution of specific disease problems that have baffled livestock owners, are made available to everyone. As a whole, it has alleviated suffering among animals, greatly reduced economic losses, helped to safeguard the livestock and food industries, and contributed to the advancement of medicine.

Origin and Spread of Important Insect Pests of Animals

Before the white man arrived in America, Stage and Hyslop point out, there had been no horses, cows, sheep, goats, or chickens on this continent for many ages. Presumably, then, the insect pests of these animals came to America along with the livestock imported by white men. Ages ago there used to be hoofed animals in America. Why did they completely disappear? Possibly the tsetse fly, not now found in this country, was responsible. A fossil tsetse fly, closely related to the insect that makes the keeping of domestic livestock impossible in extensive areas in Africa, has been found in Colorado in shale beds that go back 40 million years.

Stage and Hyslop show that insects originated the practice of "thumbing a ride" and are so expert at it that they can spread far and wide from an original center. They not only travel on their own power but drift with the wind, float on water, ride as stowaways on all sorts of conveyances (including the airplane), and in particular accompany animals and animal products everywhere. The first horn fly, an insect that does 10 million dollars, worth of damage a year, was recorded in the United States near Camden, N. J., in 1887. Ten years later it had spread throughout North America and even to Hawaii. But many insects that are serious pests abroad have not yet been introduced into the United States.

How can we prevent the introduction and spread of insects? The measures briefly discussed by these authors include quarantines, careful inspection of animals and animal products in interstate commerce, better livestock management, the introduction of natural enemies of injurious insects, and in some cases temporary removal of wild animals that may serve as hosts of certain insects.

Federal and State Regulatory Activities in Animal Disease Control

The huge and complicated livestock industry of today, which feeds millions of people and gives a livelihood to millions of farmers, handlers, tradesmen, and others is subject to a constant menace–the menace of certain diseases that can decimate herds, wipe out profits, and endanger the health and the lives of consumers. No individual acting alone could hope to meet this menace. There are diseases that can be fought only if everyone acts together, with the Federal and State Governments, to mobilize the full aid of science and put into effect such control and preventive measures as each situation demands.

This is what is back of the Federal and State regulatory activities described by Miller, Fladness, Wight, Skidmore, and Joss, of the Bureau of Animal Industry, and Moskey, of the Food and Drug Administration. The legal basis of these regulations goes back to the act of Congress that established the Bureau of Animal Industry in 1884, an amendment in 1920, another amendment in 1926, and other acts of Congress in 1890, 1903, and 1905.

The grand strategy of the fight against animal diseases has several distinct aspects. Back of all of them is constant research in the field and the laboratory to track down the causes of disease with greater and greater accuracy and discover practical safeguards, preventives, and remedies.

(1) Federal and State quarantines. The object of any quarantine is to confine a dangerous infectious disease to the smallest possible area and hold it there until it can be stamped out. By keeping imported animals under observation in quarantine, several deadly diseases have been kept out of the United States, including rinderpest, surra, and mal de caderas of horses. Drastic Federal and State quarantines have been a factor in preventing the spread of foot-and-mouth disease. Quarantines should not be imposed unless they are absolutely necessary, and they should be lifted as soon as possible.

(2) Campaigns for control and eradication. When it seems necessary and possible to wipe out a widespread disease by attacking it State by State and county by county, a long-time campaign is put into execution. The methods used depend entirely on what is most practicable in each particular case–fundamentally, that is, on the findings of the research men–the bacteriologists, parasitologists, chemists, veterinarians. In the scabies campaign, the mites that cause the disease are eradicated; in the tick fever

campaign, the ticks that carry the disease. In the dourine and the bovine tuberculosis campaigns, the infected animals have to be destroyed. In the hog cholera campaign, the animals are immunized wholesale. In the case of foot-and-mouth disease, which spreads like wildfire, swift and drastic measures are taken whenever the slightest outbreak appears, to destroy not only the affected animals but those that have been definitely exposed to infection.

(3) Public stockyards inspection. In the livestock industry today, vast numbers of animals–60 to 70 million head in a single year–are assembled at public stockyards, either for immediate slaughter or for reshipment to widely scattered areas. These crowded yards are potential centers of infection for serious diseases. The only safeguard is to man them with skilled detectors of disease who inspect so many thousands of animals day after day that they can readily spot a beast infected with diseases having visible symptoms. Among the diseases for which these men are on the lookout are anthrax, cattle and sheep scabies, tick fever, hog cholera, shipping fever, swine erysipelas, foot-and-mouth disease. Infected and exposed animals are handled as the case demands, and frequently a disease can be traced back to its local source so that the farmer can take appropriate steps. The stockyards force also supervises the necessary disinfection of premises and equipment; and in the case of animals that are to be reshipped, these men see to it that dipping for scabies, testing for Bang's disease (brucellosis) and tuberculosis, or immunizing against hog cholera are carried out.

(4) Meat inspection. The job does not end with the stockyards inspection; every animal that is to be slaughtered in the meat-packing establishments engaged in interstate commerce gets an inspection–and for most of the 70 million head, this is the second one-before it is killed; and the carcass and all its edible parts are again inspected after slaughter by white-coated veterinarians on the packing-house floor. These two inspections, of course, are primarily to safeguard the public against dangerous or objectionable meat products, but the careful records kept by the inspectors are also of great value in work on the control of animal diseases.

(5) The 28-hour law. To prevent cruelty to animals, there is a Federal law against holding them in interstate shipment for more than 28 hours in common carriers without unloading them for feed, water, and rest for a period of 5 hours. This measure has a direct relation to the health of animals, and hence to their susceptibility to disease.

(6) Regulation of biological products. A group of biological products–viruses, serums, toxins, etc.–are vitally important nowadays in combating animal diseases, just as similar products are vitally important against human diseases. Any of them that are worthless, contaminated, dangerous, harmful, or in fact anything other than they should be, can do untold damage. Hence, under Federal law, these products are regulated by the Department of Agriculture.

(7) Control of drug remedies. Drugs are somewhat similarly controlled through the laws that prohibit misbranding; these laws were tightened up by the Food, Drug, and Cosmetic Act of 1938. Insecticides are controlled under the Federal Insecticide Act. In both cases, the laws apply only to products sold outside the State in which they were manufactured.

Fighting Disease with Knowledge

There are about 8,000 veterinarians in private practice in the United States to serve the needs of some 5 million livestock owners with 200 million head of cattle, horses, swine, sheep, and goats. About 4,000 more veterinarians are engaged for the most part in various public services.

These figures, says Burch, show the necessity for keeping the public accurately and adequately informed about animal diseases. The veterinarians alone, because of their limited numbers, could not possibly do all that needs to be done. Livestock owners should be familiar with the characteristics of diseases, their dangers, and the value of sound methods in dealing with them; and this is especially true of the most serious infectious diseases and those transmissible to human beings. Veterinary practitioners, scientists, and students in training need information to keep up to date with the constant developments in this field. In short, public understanding is one of the most effective of all weapons in combating disease, whether human or animal.

Burch briefly outlines the information services and material of the Department of Agriculture in this field. Publications, extension agencies, motion pictures, lantern slides, film strips, posters, exhibits, demonstrations, public addresses, and radio broadcasts are all used. The publications include a good many intended for laymen, technical papers for veterinarians and research workers, and official reports for public officers and others. The radio performs a unique service in its ability to reach large numbers of people speedily, as in warning the public of an outbreak of foot-and-mouth disease; in dealing with such a malady even an hour saved may be important. Much worth–while educational work is also done through the personal contacts of veterinarians with farmers in the course of testing for such diseases as brucellosis and tuberculosis.

Chapter 1

LOSSES CAUSED BY ANIMAL DISEASES AND PARASITES

John R. Mohler, A.E. Wight, W.M. MacKellar, F.C. Bishopp[1]

[1] *John R. Mohler is Chief, Bureau of Animal Industry; A.E. Wight is Chief, Tuberculosis Eradication Division; W. M. MacKellar is Chief, Division of Tick Eradication and Special Diseases, Bureau of Animal Industry; and F.C. Bishopp is Assistant Chief, Bureau of Entomology and Plant Quarantine.*

Germs and Worms and other low forms of life pick close to half a billion dollars a year from the pockets of our livestock producers, often so expertly that the producer does not even realize his loss. Here are enemies that must be fought with our very best strategy, based on research.

The traditions of the oldest civilized nations show that they early recognized the importance of diseases among their animals and the danger these diseases meant to human health. Today, with a dense livestock population in many parts of the world, modern transportation facilities, and the daily concentration of large numbers of farm animals at hundreds of market centers, the opportunities for animals to become infected with diseases and parasites are greatly increased in comparison with those of the past. The prevention or control of these diseases and the protection of the public from exposure to those that are communicable to man have become complicated and costly.

The far-reaching economic consequences of animal diseases, parasites, and insects are frequently not understood or are overlooked. Most of us think little of the death of a chicken; yet the aggregate monetary loss from poultry diseases, involving mortality and non-productivity among adult fowls as well as the death of young and growing birds, is incredibly high in the course of a year. Moreover, in many cases of disease, the losses are much more extensive than the direct loss due to the death of the affected animal or the depreciation in its value. Some diseases, such as cattle tick fever, have even restricted the whole agricultural programme in the infected districts.

Some of the cost of disease prevention is chargeable to diseases that do not even exist in the United States but which in self-protection this country has to guard against by maintaining an effective quarantine service at ports of entry. The communicability to man of a number of animal diseases is well known, and this danger adds to the economic losses. The need for and the cost of meat and milk inspection are in large part due to the necessity of guarding the consumer against animal diseases that may be transmitted by these food products. Quarantines within our own country, which either prevent or restrict the movement of animals from a specified area, are important and necessary control measures, but generally they adversely affect the value of the healthy as well as the diseased animals within the quarantined area; and sometimes, as in an area quarantined on account of cattle tick infestation, even the land values may depreciate. For protection against other diseases, such as hog cholera, anthrax, and encephalomyelitis, enormous numbers of healthy animals have to be immunized each year. In addition to the monetary losses from contagious and infectious diseases, there are those resulting from sporadic diseases, poisonous plants, wounds, and injuries, which, taken together, amount to a very large sum. In fact, it has been estimated that the loss solely from shipping injuries to food-producing animals due to abuse, carelessness, or other preventable causes amounts to at least 11.5 million dollars annually.

The intangible or indirect nature of much of the loss due to animal diseases makes it impossible to calculate the exact amount in dollars and cents. However, it has been estimated to be nearly one-half of a billion dollars annually. In the never-ending fight to reduce this drain on the livestock industry, hundreds of scientific workers are constantly employed, both publicly and privately. Large sums are expended each year by the States and the Federal Government for the prevention, control, and eradication of diseases now present in the United States and to guard against the introduction of new diseases and pests from abroad.

The following examples of a few of the more important diseases and pests will serve to show the extent of some of these losses.

Tuberculosis

The existence of tuberculosis among farm animals causes serious losses, partly because the disease is communicable between different classes of livestock. Swine, for example, readily contract the avian type of tuberculosis when exposed to poultry infected with the disease, and the susceptibility of human beings to tuberculosis of the bovine type has an important bearing on public health problems.

Much progress has been made in the control and eradication of tuberculosis in livestock during the last 24 years, as evidenced by the great reduction in the percentage of cattle that react to the tuberculin test and by the reduction in the number of carcasses and parts of carcasses condemned for this disease at slaughtering establishments operating under Federal inspection. During the fiscal year 1941 approximately 12,229,500 tuberculin tests were applied to cattle by veterinarians under the direction of the officials conducting cooperative tuberculosis-eradication work. The percentage of cattle that reacted to these tests was 0.3, the lowest average degree of infection found in any year since the work was undertaken in 1917. The percentage that year was approximately 5, while the annual financial loss from bovine tuberculosis alone was conservatively estimated at 25 million dollars. Also during 1917 slightly more than 2 percent of all the cattle slaughtered in establishments operating under Federal supervision were retained for further inspection because some evidence of tuberculosis was shown on post-mortem examination. About 195,500 cattle carcasses were retained, of which about 41,000 were condemned as unfit for human food. On the other hand, during the fiscal year ended June 30, 1941, the percentage of cattle retained, exclusive of known reactors to the tuberculin test, was 0.07. About 8,000 cattle carcasses were retained, of which 1,584 were condemned as unfit for human food.

During the fiscal year 1917, evidence of tuberculosis was reported in approximately 10 percent of all the hogs slaughtered under Federal supervision, and about 168,000 carcasses, or 0.41 percent of the number slaughtered, were condemned as unfit for food or passed for sterilization. The percentage of retentions increased gradually up to 1924, when it was 15.2, an increase of about 50 per cent during that period of 7 years. Since 1924 the percentage of retentions has gradually diminished; during the fiscal year 1941 it was 8.2, and the number of carcasses condemned and sterilized was 31,200, or 0.06 percent of the number slaughtered. Much of the tuberculosis now being reported in swine is of the avian type.

The cooperative tuberculosis-eradication work among livestock has consisted largely in the tuberculin testing of cattle and the removal of reactors to the test. Through the combined efforts of all State, Federal, and county livestock officials, breeders, dairymen, and others, it was possible to apply about 241,950,000 tuberculin tests to cattle in this country from 1917 to June 30, 1941; about 3,809,000 reactors were disclosed and disposed of for slaughter. All the counties in all the States had qualified as modified accredited tuberculosis-free areas on November 1, 1940, indicating that the disease was present in less than one-half of 1 percent of the cattle population.

The losses caused by tuberculosis in poultry are considerable each year, especially in 11 of the North Central States, owing to mortality, decreased egg production, and general unthriftiness.

Other Diseases

Brucellosis exists among cattle to some extent in all parts of the United States, but it is much more prevalent in some localities than in others.

Considerable research work on the control of this disease had been accomplished in this country before 1934, and in some States quite a large number of herds of cattle had been freed of it. In 1934 a cooperative eradication plan was put into effect. At that time it was estimated that approximately 10 percent of the dairy and breeding cattle over 6 months of age in this country would react to the blood-agglutination test used to diagnose the disease, and many writers estimated that the annual loss due to the disease from reduction in the calf crop, non-breeding, and reduction in milk production was in the neighborhood of 50 million dollars. Many breeders of purebred cattle, who had spent a lifetime building up herds with animals of irreplaceable blood lines, were forced out of business by the presence of a virulent type of the disease.

Since 1934 the incidence of infection with brucellosis has been considerably reduced. A large number of herds have passed three tests showing no infection within a period of a year and have qualified as accredited brucellosis-free herds. Also, a considerable number of counties have qualified as modified accredited areas, indicating that in county-wide testing of all the dairy and breeding cattle over 6 months of age, not more than 1 percent of the cattle or 5 percent of the herds were found to be infected. In many of these counties the degree of infection is less than 1 percent.

Johne's disease, which affects ruminants principally, was identified in this country probably 35 or 40 years ago. The causative agent, a bacillus, is expelled through body excretions and can be easily spread from farm to farm in many ways, the most important of which, no doubt, is by the introduction of infected cattle into clean herds.

It is difficult to estimate the monetary losses due to Johne's disease, as it probably exists unreported in many localities. On the basis of information from various reliable sources, however, it is believed that the financial losses are approximately half a million dollars a year. The disease has not been reported in human beings, although medical authorities have reported a chronic dysentery with symptoms similar to those found in cattle affected with Johne's disease. No satisfactory treatment for the disease is known at present.

Cattle tick fever was once the most serious obstacle faced by the cattle owners of the South. During the last half of the nineteenth century cattle died from it by the thousands, and at the beginning of this century it was estimated to be taking an annual toll of 40 million dollars from the South. All attempts at medicinal treatment had proved ineffective in controlling these losses. Following the discovery that the cattle tick was the only natural carrier of the disease, however, it became evident that without the tick the disease would be of little importance and would probably die out. On this theory efforts to eradicate the cattle tick were undertaken in 1906 and have continued uninterruptedly up to the present time, with the result that the area quarantined for cattle tick fever has been reduced to about 1 percent of its original size and the disease is no longer considered a serious menace in the United States.

Probably no other infectious animal disease is so widespread as hog cholera, and few parts of the world where swine are grown are free from its ravages. Since the first report of its appearance in Ohio in 1833, it has spread to every State in the Union. During certain years, notably 1887, 1897, 1913, and 1926, the disease seemed to flare up in a virulent form and was unusually widespread in the United States, with estimated monetary losses amounting to 65 million dollars for a single year. In recent years the extensive immunization of swine with anti-hog-cholera serum and virus has held losses to a lower level, but notwithstanding these extensive prophylactic measures Log cholera continues to be the most serious and destructive disease of swine. It is estimated that directly and indirectly the disease is still responsible for an average annual loss of about 12.5 million dollars to the swine growers of the country.

Parasites and Other Pests

The losses from the depredations of parasites affect not only the producers of livestock but also the meat industry and some other industries that utilize certain animal products for commercial purposes. The greatest losses, however, are sustained by livestock producers in the form of unthriftiness in stock, debility usually associated with digestive and respiratory disturbances, stunting, and death of young stock and poultry. The unhealthiness in particular is a serious drain on the resources of livestock producers, since it involves the expenditure of rather large sums of money for medication to alleviate symptoms of sickness as well as waste of feed in unsuccessful attempts to promote growth and fattening of parasitized animals.

It is difficult to estimate the death losses from parasites because there is no machinery for collecting information of this sort. That such losses are considerable, however, is evident from the fact that parasitism in livestock and poultry is widespread in this country; that severe death losses, sometimes as great as 10 percent, occur quite frequently among all classes of stock and poultry; that the losses have been reduced sharply in special cases by resorting to control measures and effective medication; that it is the common experience of sheep producers that lambs cannot be raised successfully on the farm without resorting to periodic drenching or other treatment with medicinal preparations and without making provision for rotation or other methods of parasite control; and that successful swine husbandry involves a special system of management designed to hold in check infections with roundworms, lungworms, kidney worms, and the other parasites that are responsible for most of the unthriftiness and stunting so common in pigs in many parts of this country.

The losses due to unthriftiness and stunting are even more difficult to estimate than the actual death losses. It is known, however, from information published by various investigators, that the waste of feed in raising and fattening parasitized stock must be enormous. For instance, it has been determined that whereas an average of 3.1 pounds of feed produced a gain of 1 pound in 7 weeks in chicks protected from parasites, 4.5 pounds of feed was required to produce this gain in weight in parasitized birds. In extensive studies conducted some years ago on 150 farms in the Middle West on which effective parasite control for swine was practiced, it was found that pigs with which these special precautions were taken were ready for market 7 weeks younger than the average age at which pigs in that area were usually marketed, and that at 4 months of age the pigs so protected weighed 28 pounds more than pigs that had become parasitized. In a recent study by parasitologists of the Bureau of Animal Industry it was determined that sheep that acquired even a moderate infection with nodular worms on a pasture over a period of several months weighed on an average 10 pounds less than comparable sheep on a similar pasture free from nodular worm larvae.

The losses sustained by the meat industry have been ascertained much more extensively and accurately than those occurring on the farm. In large sections of the South where pigs are commonly affected with kidney worms the average loss per pig due to condemnation of the liver, kidneys, and kidney fat and trimming of loins to remove worms and lesions is nearly 40 cents a head. Several years ago it was estimated that the losses due to the condemnation of sheep intestines (used for casings and in the preparation of surgical suture material) because of pathological conditions produced by nodular worms amounted to about $200,000 in one State. The annual loss on beef and sheep livers condemned under meat inspection because of parasitic infestations of various kinds may be conservatively estimated at half a million dollars a year.

In spite of the general paucity of information on which to base accurate figures, it may be estimated conservatively that the total losses from parasites of all kinds, including the cost of drugs to keep these pests in check and the labour and equipment involved in special systems of management for controlling them, are about 125 million dollars a year. Of this large total, it is estimated that the diseases due to protozoan parasites, of which coccidiosis is of greatest economic importance, exact an annual toll from the resources of farmers, stockmen, and poultrymen of about 10 million dollars, half of which is chargeable to poultry coccidiosis. Furthermore, the combined losses from liver flukes in cattle, sheep, and goats and from tapeworms in all classes of stock and poultry are estimated at 5 million dollars a year. The large bulk of the remaining loss (about 110 million dollars) is chargeable to nematodes, or roundworms.

Insects, mites, and ticks are responsible for tremendous losses among livestock of all kinds. Many of these pests act as disease transmitters, most of them carrying diseases accidentally. Some serve as intermediate hosts of diseases organisms, that is, the organisms must pass through an essential cycle of development in the body of the insect. Insects damage livestock directly by causing loss of blood or destruction of tissue, and they irritate and worry the animals by their presence or their bites. The resulting losses take the form of increased mortality, lowered general condition, slower growth, increased, feed consumption, lowered work output, and reduced quantity and quality of such products as milk, wool, and hides.

The constant and persistent attacks of such pests as horn flies, stableflies, and horseflies, and, to some extent, mosquitoes produce nervous reactions that often cause grazing animals to stop feeding and seek such shelter as may be found in streams and shady places.

Under such circumstances it is impossible for them to put on flesh, and consequently it is difficult to bring them to a marketable condition. In dairy animals there is a direct loss due to lowered milk flow. Death is sometimes caused by concentrated attacks of particularly vicious species. The buffalo gnat is notorious in some of the Southern States for its destruction of animals, especially mules.

Mosquitoes cause heavier losses among livestock than is generally realized. For the most part the losses are more or less intangible and incapable of being appraised in terms of dollars and cents; they are due chiefly to interference with the normal development and well-being of the animals. Along the Gulf coast cattle are frequently driven from their feeding grounds in the marshes into the open water by mosquito attacks. Deaths of cattle from the concentrated attack of the large mosquito (*Psorophora columbiae*) are a matter of record.

The common housefly annoys all classes of livestock by crawling about on them and feeding on the secretions of the eyes and body openings. It also is capable of transmitting certain diseases of livestock, such as mastitis. What is more important, this fly may contaminate milk and other dairy products with the germs of such human diseases as typhoid, dysentery, tuberculosis, and cholera.

The most extensive losses to the livestock industry caused by insects are those due to the attacks of species that penetrate the living tissues of the animal and derive their entire sustenance during their period of growth from the body of their host. Some of these, such as the cattle grub, or heel fly, the horse bot, and the head bot of sheep, spend the greater part of the year within the body of the host animal. All three of these insects occasionally attack man and penetrate the body or head tissues. They cause much suffering and make medical attention necessary.

The damage wrought by screwworms and blowflies on livestock is spectacular, and the losses are all too apparent. The primary screwworm will attack any animal on which there is an injury, however slight. Thousands of cases of screwworm injury occur each year in the South and especially the Southwest. The cost of treatment, added to the value of animals killed by screwworms each year, constitutes a very heavy loss, which has been estimated to be at least 5 million dollars annually in the United States.

Lice of various species attack practically all the domestic animals and cause varying degrees of loss. Goat lice retard the development of young goats, lower the quality of mohair, reduce the amount of the clip, and frequently cause death. Chicken lice reduce egg production to a marked degree and lower the vitality of the fowls. Mites, fowl ticks, and sticktight fleas supplement the attacks of lice on chickens, and the combined result is a heavy loss to the poultry industry. The loss caused by the attacks of lice on cattle, horses, and hogs is less tangible but no less real. At the least a heavy infestation means decreased vitality.

Mites producing scabies or mange are the source of varying degrees of loss. In sheep, infestations of scab mites result in the loss of large quantities of wool by shedding, and heavy infestations may so weaken the animals that they may die. Mange mites produce an unhealthy condition in other animals which in extreme cases may destroy their usefulness. The expense of enforcing quarantines against scab and mange is by no means a small item. Fortunately losses in this country from these mites have been greatly reduced in recent years by dipping operations.

Certain insects and allied classes of arthropods, such as ticks, transmit diseases to animals and are thus chargeable with the losses caused by these diseases. Outstanding in this group is the cattle tick, which transmits tick, or splenetic, fever of cattle. Anthrax is transmitted from animal to animal by biting flies and may be transmitted to man in the same way. Anaplasmosis is likewise transmitted by ticks and certain insects, and equine encephalomyelitis has been shown to be transmitted by mosquitoes. Buffalo gnats transmit the leucocytozoan disease of wild and tame ducks and a similar disease of turkeys. In Michigan some severe losses of ducks have occurred, and apparently heavy losses among young turkeys result from this malady.

Various parasitic worms of animals pass an essential stage of their existence in the bodies of insects. Without the insects as intermediate hosts they would never reach the stage where they can become animal parasites.

Finally, insects that destroy forage are responsible for considerable loss of livestock feed. The devastation of ranges by grasshoppers within the last few years has cut rather deeply into the profits from stock raising in the affected regions.

A Tabulation of Losses

A conservative estimate of annual losses from the more important diseases, parasites, and pests of livestock and poultry, as of January 1, 1942, is included in the following tabulation:

Item	Loss
Internal parasites	$125,000,000
External parasites of poultry	85,000,000
Cattle grubs	65,000,000
Poultry diseases (except tuberculosis and those caused by parasites)	40,000,000
Brucellosis of cattle (Bang's disease)	30,000,000
Mastitis	19,000,000
Hog cholera	12,500,000
Tuberculosis (cattle, swine, and poultry)	10,500,000
Swine abortion	10,000,000
Stablefly and horn fly	10,000,000
Screwworms	5,000,000
Cattle and sheep scabies	1,000,000
Encephalomyelitis	1,000,000
Swine erysipelas	1,000,000
Anthrax	750,000
Johne's disease	500,000
Hemorrhagic septicemia	500,000
Goat lice	500,000
Cattle tick fever	400,000
Rabies	250,000
Anaplasmosis	100,000
Total	$418,000,000

Chapter 2

CAUSES OF DISEASES

H.W. Schoening, Benjamin Schwartz, Ward T. Huffman, and Louis L. Madsen[1]

[1] *H.W. Schoening, Chief, Pathological Division, Bureau of Animal Industry, prepared the introductory statement and the section on Bacterial and Virus Infections; Benjamin Schwartz, Chief, Zoological Division, Bureau of Animal Industry, prepared the material on Animal Parasites; Ward T. Huffman, in Charge of Stock Poisoning Caused by Plants, Pathological Division, Bureau of Animal Industry, at Salt Lake City, Utah, wrote Poisonous Plants as Causes of Disease; and Louis L. Madsen, Nutritionist, Animal Nutrition Division Bureau of Animal Industry, contributed the section on Nutritional Deficiencies as Causes of Diseases.*

This article gives basic information about bacteria, viruses, and internal parasites–what they are, what they do to the body, and how they do it–and includes brief discussions of nutritional deficiencies and plant poisons as two other important causes of disease in livestock.

The animal body is composed of an intricate, coordinated collection of cells of various types, bound together by connecting tissues. The outer layer of all the tissues together is the common covering, the skin. The cells that make up the various tissues have specific functions to perform, and a certain interdependence of all the tissues and functions is necessary for the maintenance of health. Any agent that is inimical to the life and functions of the cells and tissues may be considered a disease-producing agent, and disease may be defined as any abnormal condition of the tissues of the body.

Among disease-producing agents may be mentioned germs, viruses, parasites (internal and external), chemicals, poisons of various kinds, faulty nutrition, and injuries.

In a broad sense, a disease process can be considered as an inflammation. The suffix "itis" means "inflammation of," and when attached to the root of the name of an anatomical part, it means an inflammation of that part; examples are appendicitis, an inflammation of the appendix; tonsillitis, an inflammation of the tonsils; and peritonitis, an inflammation of the peritoneum, the abdominal lining membrane. Whatever the factor that causes disease may be and wherever it may be located in the body its activities result in an inflammation of the part affected. Any injury results in the destruction of tissues and cells, and the inflammatory reaction that follows is an effort on the part of the body to repair the injury. The effort is manifested by an increased circulation to the part affected and the seepage of serum and other blood elements into the tissues for the purpose of removing the damaged tissue. The ability of the body to repair the damage caused by the disease-producing agent determines, whether or not the affected part will recover, or return to its normal state.

In this article, infection with bacteria, viruses, and parasites, poisoning by plants, and nutritional deficiencies will be considered as factors in the production of disease.

Bacterial and Virus Infections

Infections that cause disease are the result of invasion of the tissues by micro-organisms (bacteria) or viruses. These agents gain entrance to the animal body in various ways through the respiratory, digestive, and genital tracts and the skin, and they then multiply and attack the tissues, producing a disease condition. This is not readily accomplished, however, for the body forces make strenuous efforts to repel the invaders. The mechanism of infection and resistance is quite complex. The two factors primarily concerned are the disease-producing agent and the animal itself (the host). For an infecting agent to invade the tissues of a host successfully, it must have sufficient virulence (ability to overcome the body defences) to establish itself within the host's body, and then it must be able either to multiply actively, producing a disease process, or to survive in a quiescent state (the carrier stage) until conditions are right for multiplication or it escapes from the host and becomes infectious to other susceptible animals. The host, on the other hand, is protected, within limits, by the barrier known as immunity or resistance. Generally speaking, resistance is relative, and varies considerably among individual animals. In some it may be quite strong; in others, weak or entirely lacking.

The infective agent is greatly influenced by its surroundings, either within or outside the animal host. Its invading ability is determined to a large extent by the environment. It is well known that certain species of animals are highly resistant to certain types of infection; the resistance of cattle to glanders, a disease of horses, may be cited as an example. In the species susceptible to a specific infection, however, there will also be found a wide variation in susceptibility and resistance among individuals. Resistance (immunity) to a disease process may be built up in certain animals to an appreciable extent by natural contact with limited amounts of infection in the field that do not produce a frank expression of the disease, and also by artificial procedures such as vaccination. It should be noted, however, that there is a wide variation in the immunity response of individual animals to the same vaccination procedure. It is not possible to say at present just what makes one animal more resistant to infection than another; it may be that a number of factors, either singly or in combination, are involved.

The success achieved in breeding plants resistant to certain diseases is well known. That heredity prays a part in some, at least, of the disease processes in animals is also known. Experimental work on cancer of mice has shown the part heredity can play in this disease, and evidence has been found in studies of bursati, or summer sores, in horses that the primary causative factor is a genetic one.

Other factors to be considered are nutrition, the influence of the glands of internal secretion, and even management practices. Recent experiments have shown that the diet of pregnant mice and actively growing young mice has a considerable influence on the resistance of these animals to invasion by a virus affecting the nervous system. Hereditary, physiological, nutritional, and management factors may all play an important part in the development of disease.

Bacteria as Disease-Producing Agents

Bacteria, or germs, are microscopic organisms of various sizes and shapes. They are found everywhere in nature. Though some of them are capable of producing disease, many more are not only harmless but are of actual benefit through their activity in changing the composition of substances–for example, those that create the fermentation processes used in the manufacture of vinegar and the ripening of cheese. Bacteria capable of producing disease are known as pathogens, or pathogenic bacteria; those that do not produce disease are known as saprophytes, or nonpathogens.

During the last 50 years tremendous advances have been made in the science of bacteriology, and large numbers of micro-organisms have been identified as either causing specific diseases or being associated with a disease process. A system of classification has been developed whereby these microscopic organisms are identified and placed in various groups. In this article, the term "bacteria" is used in its broad sense to include all the various classes of micro-organisms that cause disease.

Bacteria are of various sizes and shapes and have distinguishing, features by which they can be identified. It has been possible to grow them on artificial media in test tubes, and through various laboratory techniques it is possible to study pure strains of the organisms. The ability of various bacteria to utilize certain food substances is a further aid in differentiation. Some bacteria grow only in the presence of oxygen, others only in the complete absence of oxygen, and a third group with or without oxygen.

Some bacteria are actively motile; their physical make-up enables them to move about swiftly in the proper media. Others do not have this power of locomotion and are spoken of as non-motile.

Some bacteria are capable under certain circumstances of forming spores. As spores, they are in a resting stage during which they are highly resistant to adverse influences, such as heat and the action of disinfectants, and may remain alive for years.

Some bacteria are able to produce powerful poisons, known as soluble toxins, in the medium in which they grow. Other bacteria carry toxins within their bodies which are liberated and exert their action when the bacteria are broken up. These, which are known as endotoxins, are not as powerful as the soluble toxins. Diseases such as tetanus (lockjaw) and diphtheria are caused by bacteria that produce powerful soluble toxins.

Further studies of pathogenic bacteria can be made through their disease-producing action on laboratory animals, such as rabbits, guinea pigs, and mice, when they are introduced into these animals by injection, feeding, or through contact exposure.

Certain diseases are produced by specific bacteria. The bacteria that cause diseases are of various types and classes, and the diseases they produce and their methods of spread are also quite varied.

Certain types of bacteria produce localized inflammatory changes in tissues, such as abscesses. Depending on the virulence of the organism and the resistance of the animal, these abscesses may remain localized, or the infection may enter the blood stream and cause a serious general disturbance and sometimes death from septicemia.

The Filtrable Viruses

In addition to diseases produced by bacteria, there are others caused by filtrable viruses. A virus may be defined as an infectious agent capable of passing through filters that retain bacteria. The viruses are ultramicroscopic, that is, they cannot be seen under the highest powered microscope. Among the animal diseases caused by viruses are foot-and-mouth disease, hog cholera, rabies, equine encephalomyelitis, fowl pox, and laryngotracheitis of poultry. Smallpox, measles, influenza, and mumps are examples of virus diseases of man. To date, more than 35 virus diseases of animals have been identified and studied.

The virus diseases have come into special prominence in the past few years, and as a result of a vast amount of experimental work in various countries of the world, knowledge concerning them has increased considerably. Exact information on the nature of viruses is not available. They have been considered to be living entities, although recent work indicates that some of them may not be living but that they may be able to produce a substance that acts as a catalytic agent and causes cell injury. This work has been principally in the field of plant viruses, and no evidence has yet been produced to indicate that animal viruses are not living agents. Although for many years bacteria have been grown on artificial media and this process has provided an excellent opportunity to increase our knowledge concerning these organisms and the part they play in the production of disease, it has not been possible until recently to cultivate the viruses in artificial media. It is necessary that media for viruses contain living cells. The use of tissue cultures has made it possible for certain viruses to be carried indefinitely through regular transfers.

In addition to growing the viruses on tissue culture, it has also been possible to propagate many of them in growing chick embryos by methods developed through studies begun in 1931. Through certain technical procedures, an opening is made in the eggshell, and suitable material containing the virus is inoculated in the membranes surrounding the embryo. The virus multiplies in the living cells and produces pathological changes in the membranes or the embryo or both.

Through these recently developed methods of propagating viruses, it has been possible to obtain much information on their physical and chemical properties, and this has resulted in the development of immunization methods for the control of many virus diseases. Not all the disease-producing viruses have been grown on artificial media, however. Just why it has been possible to grow some and not others is not yet known, and much research work is still needed to obtain additional information on this subject.

The viruses that cause diseases of animals may be classified for the purposes of study and discussion according to the tissues they invade. Thus, the virus diseases are sometimes spoken of as neurotropic, epitheliotropic, and viscerotropic, which means that they attack principally neuron, or nerve, tissue (nerves, brain, spinal cord, etc.), epithelial tissue (skin and membranes), or visceral tissue (many or all internal tissues).

Some diseases produced by viruses are confined principally to certain tissues, but others, though affecting a certain type of tissue primarily, may also involve other tissues. The division indicated is, therefore, quite arbitrary but is used as a basis for discussion.

Secondary Bacterial Invaders

Certain of the virus diseases are often complicated by the action of so-called secondary bacterial invaders. These are bacteria that may be normally present in the animal without harm or may be responsible for a low-grade infection that is of no serious consequence but becomes active and capable of invading the tissues to produce severe disease complications following a virus infection. A vicious circle may be established by the virus and the secondary bacterial infection, the action of one increasing the virulence of the other, with disastrous effects. This often occurs in distemper of dogs and horses, swine influenza, hog cholera, and other virus diseases.

How Diseases are Transmitted

Once established in a susceptible animal, as already noted, the infectious agent attacks certain tissues, multiplies, and sets up a disease process. Quantities of the causative agent are eliminated in various ways by the infected animal through its secretions and excretions so that its surroundings become contaminated. Susceptible animals coming in contact with the contagion thus have an opportunity to become infected. The ability of the infection to survive outside an animal body until it is able to gain entrance to a new host determines to a large extent its disease-spreading ability.

Biting insects, such as flies and mosquitoes, and other pests, such as ticks, are capable of transmitting and do transmit specific infections from infected to healthy animals under proper conditions.

In diseases such as tuberculosis the contagious matter is eliminated with the secretions and excretions of the animal. The surroundings become contaminated, and susceptible animals coming in contact with material that is still active can readily become infected. On the other hand, exposure to sunlight, dryness, or similar conditions over a suitable period of time has an adverse effect on the viability of the organism and its ability to invade susceptible animals.

Certain bacteria can live for indefinite periods outside the animal body and still retain a high degree of virulence. An outstanding example of this is the anthrax organism. In the final stages of the disease in an animal, the blood stream and all the tissues contain large quantities of the organisms in what is known as a vegetative stage. When these vegetative forms become exposed to the air through the opening of the carcass or the escape of blood from the natural openings of the body, they develop into spores. In this stage the organisms are extremely difficult to kill. They can withstand high and low temperatures and have been known to retain their infective capacity for years. It can therefore be seen that once soil becomes infected with anthrax spores it may remain dangerous for susceptible animals for long periods of time.

Another disease-producing organism that is quite resistant to adverse influences is the germ causing swine erysipelas. While this organism does not go into a spore stage, it can live in certain soils for long periods, and the suggestion has even been made that active multiplication may take place in suitable types of soil. Here again the infected animal contaminates its surroundings through its discharges.

Although the virus diseases have certain things in common, their mode of transmission may vary considerably, depending on the nature of the disease and the extent to which the virus has multiplied within the body of the affected animal. Infection takes place when the virus in a proper state is introduced into a susceptible animal.

Rabies and equine encephalomyelitis may be mentioned as examples of the neurotropic virus diseases of animals.

Rabies is caused by a filtrable virus which is found in the saliva of an animal affected with the disease and is transmitted under natural conditions through the bite of a rabid animal, usually a dog. The disease results in degenerative changes in the brain which cause affected animals to become aggressive and attack or bite any available object. After the virus is deposited in the tissues, usually through the injury made by the bite, it is considered that it moves from the site of deposit by way of the nerves, eventually reaching the central nervous system the brain and spinal cord. The symptoms of the disease, which terminates finally, then develop.

Equine encephalomyelitis, sometimes known as sleeping sickness or blind staggers of horses, is another virus disease that attacks principally the brain and spinal cord, although experimentally it has also been found capable of propagating in other tissues, including those of the skin. Early in the infection the virus of equine encephalomyelitis is found for a short time in the blood stream. It then disappears from the blood and is found only in the brain and spinal cord. Nervous symptoms of the disease are noted early. It has been shown experimentally that this disease can be transmitted by the bites of a number of different species of mosquitoes and other insects. The virus of the western type has been isolated from mosquitoes (*Culex tarsalis*) found in nature and also from the assassin bug (*Triatoma sanguisuga*). The disease is therefore considered to be spread chiefly through biting insects.

Foot-and-mouth disease is an example of an epitheliotropic virus. Although not now present in the United States, it has been one of the chief animal scourges for many years in other parts of the world. In addition to being one of the most important, if not the most important, of the animal diseases, it has particular interest in this discussion because it was the first animal disease shown to be caused by a filtrable virus. This was accomplished in 1898 through the research work of two German investigators, Loeffler and Frosch.

The vesicles, which contain the infective agent, break, and the virus is thus disseminated in the litter and on the ground where susceptible animals coming in contact with it easily pick up the infection. In the early stages of the disease the blood itself is infectious, and it has been shown that at that time the milk, the saliva, the urine, and also the feces may contain the virus. Because of the large quantities of the virus eliminated by affected animals and is highly infectious nature, a wide dissemination of the disease within a comparatively short time is possible.

Carriers of Disease and Reservoirs of Viruses

In addition to the transmission of disease from a sick animal to a normal one, either by direct contact or through contamination of the surroundings with the disease-producing agent, disease may be transmitted by another means, namely, by the carrier animal.

A carrier animal is one that carries an infective agent within its body without showing appreciable evidence of illness. The infective agent may be eliminated from time to time and act as a source of infection to other animals; or the carrier animal itself through some adverse condition may develop a frank attack of the disease; or the infection may be carried from a carrier to a normal animal through the bite of an insect.

It has been believed for many years that certain animals that have recovered from infection with the virus of foot-and-mouth disease may retain active virus within their bodies over a period of months and even years, eliminating it from time to time in sufficient quantities to produce the disease in susceptible animals. The virus might be enclosed in the growing hoof as the result of infection of the coronary band, escaping when the growth of the hoof reaches a certain stage; or it might rest in some part of the body in an inactive state and later be eliminated in the secretions or excretions of the animal.

In infectious anemia of horses–so-called swamp fever–a carrier stage is seen in which an apparently normal animal carries the infective agent in its blood stream for many years, perhaps during the rest of its life. It appears from the available evidence that this disease is transmitted principally by biting insects.

When animals or birds of a wide variety of species are susceptible to a common infection, an individual of one of the species may be a carrier or reservoir of the disease from which infection may be spread to other susceptible species through insect bites. For example, a large number of avian species have been found experimentally to be susceptible to equine encephalomyelitis, and the pigeon and ring-necked pheasant have been found to be affected with this disease in nature. Other laboratory tests indicate that other birds and mammals may harbour the infection. It is considered quite probable that birds may act as reservoirs of the virus to a greater extent than horses and other mammals and that infection may be carried from infected birds to a variety of susceptible species by mosquitoes and other biting insects.

Animal Parasites

As used in this book, the term "parasites" refers to low forms of animal life that live on or in other animals larger than themselves. An animal that harbours parasites is known as a host. Some parasites require only one host for the completion of their life cycles, whereas others require more than one. In the former case the life cycle is direct; in the latter, it is indirect. The host in which a parasite develops to maturity is known as the final, or definitive, host; that in which only the parasite's larval (immature) stages develop is called the intermediate host. As a rule, hosts are more or less seriously affected by their parasites, the injury suffered depending on the kinds and, usually, the numbers of parasites harboured.

When parasites invade a host in numbers sufficient to produce injury to health, they set up an infection, which is designated as a parasitic infection to differentiate it from infections produced by bacteria or viruses. There is no absolute dividing line, however, between infections caused by parasites and those caused by other living agents. Bacteria multiply within the host, as do many parasites also. Most of the larger parasites that do not increase in number within the host increase greatly in size. In both instances there is multiplication of foreign cells within the host.

Parasites have played an important role in the history of civilization, because they cause many of the ills to which human beings and animals are subject. Certain parts of the world are unsuited for civilization largely because of the prevalence in those regions of parasitic diseases that injure and destroy human life and domestic animals. Many areas that were formerly unsuitable for civilized living, however, have been made safe, in whole or in part, by the vigourous application of sanitary measures designed to keep parasitic diseases in check or to eradicate them.

Malaria, one of the most deadly diseases of mankind, African sleeping sickness, and amoebic dysentery are examples of devastating human parasitic diseases caused by micro-organisms known as protozoa. Diseases more or less closely related to them occur also in domestic animals and poultry. Hookworm disease, at one time an important factor in the physical and mental retardation of a considerable portion of the population of the southern part of the United States, and still a public health problem of considerable importance in the tropical and subtropical belts of the globe, including parts of this country, is an outstanding example of a dangerous worm infection. Hookworms and related bloodsucking parasites occur in all kinds of domestic animals, producing injuries essentially similar to those observed in infected human beings. In short, parasites are capable of adversely affecting the health of animals as well as of man and of producing debilitating diseases that may result in death.

If all the parasites to which man and domestic animals are subject were equally injurious, the human and livestock populations would have been decimated long ago. Of the hundreds of species of parasitic organisms that find a haven on or in the bodies of human beings, animals, and birds, some are far more injurious than others, and many inflict more or less injury without actually producing a distinct disease. Unlike the diseases caused by bacteria and viruses, which appear suddenly with almost explosive violence and are accompanied by prostration and high fever, many of those produced by parasites tend to be chronic and are not accompanied by fever. Parasitic infections of many types are characterized by stunted growth, emaciation, general unthriftiness, digestive disturbances, and gradual wasting. Even when such infections are only moderate, deaths may occur here and there; but as a rule there is nothing comparable to the wholesale mortality that takes place, in outbreaks of infectious diseases such as anthrax or hog cholera. Because of their insidious nature, however, some parasitic infections may take a rather severe toll from the resources of farmers and stockmen before the presence of the offending organisms in a herd is even suspected. The stealthy march of parasitism, in contrast to the open approach of infectious diseases, sometimes makes the former the deadlier of the two.

Hundreds of different kinds of parasites affect human beings, livestock, and poultry. Thousands of others occur in various wild animals, birds, fishes, and other forms of animal life. Many of the parasites of domestic animals and poultry occur also in wild animals and birds. In some cases parasites of one kind of domestic animal are transmissible to other kinds of domestic animals. Certain parasites of animals are transmissible to man, and vice versa. In view of the diversity of parasitic organisms and their range in host relationships, it is essential to classify parasites on the basis of their natural relationships and, for the sake of convenience, also with reference to their adaptability to various hosts.

Under the designation of parasites are included a number of animal groups, some of which are only remotely related to one another. In fact parasitism is so widespread in the animal kingdom that very few of the major groups of animals are altogether free from forms that lead a parasitic existence. Fortunately, however, from the standpoint of human and animal health only three groups need be taken into consideration: (1) Protozoa, or unicellular animals, (2) worms, or helminths, and (3) insects, ticks, and related forms, known as arthropods, many of which act as intermediate hosts and vectors for infective parasites.

Protozoa

Protozoa, or protozoans, are the simplest forms of animal life, the entire body of one of these organisms consisting of a single cell.

The protozoans are thus differentiated from all other animals, which are designated as metazoans (many-celled animals). Protozoans were first discovered during the latter part of the seventeenth century by Leeuwenhoek in Holland, who constructed the simple microscopes that he used in their discovery. This man of genius, known as the inventor of the microscope and the discoverer of micro-organisms, investigated, among other things, stagnant water and the intestinal contents of various animals. He even made studies on himself, thereby discovering human parasitic protozoans.

Since Leeuwenhoek's day an ever-growing army of investigators has studied protozoan organisms, some of which are free-living and occur in fresh, brackish, and salt water, in soil, and in a variety of other locations. Other protozoans are not free-living but parasitic in various parts of the bodies of animals of all kinds, including human beings. With the exception of a few that are within the limits of unaided vision, the vast majority of protozoans can be seen only through the microscope. Certain protozoans, particularly among those that are parasitic, are so small that they must be studied with the highest magnification available.

Some groups of parasitic protozoans resemble more or less closely related free-living forms, whereas others contain only parasitic species. The latter (sporozoans) have become so greatly modified by the parasitic mode of life that they have no organs of locomotion. Some protozoans (amoebae), move by a flowing of the entire body substance, others (flagellates) by means of one or more whiplike lashes known as flagella, and some (ciliates) by small vibratile processes, called cilia, located all over the body. Protozoans of all four groups occur in man and animals, and some of them produce serious and fatal diseases.

Many protozoans multiply by simple division, the entire body dividing into two parts, each a more or less exact duplicate of the other. The two individuals that result from simple division become separated, and each leads an independent existence. The process of division is repeated many times, until eventually a host that originally acquired only a few of the organisms may be teeming with them. In other protozoans multiple division takes place, the body dividing in succession into a number of similar parts, each of which finally grows into a form like the parent organism. Since each of these organisms is capable sooner or later of repeating the process of multiple division, they can overwhelm the host in a comparatively short time. Parasitic amoebae and flagellates that live in man, domestic animals, and poultry multiply by simple division, as do also ciliates parasitic in man and animals. Some of the sporozoans, however, including malarial organisms, coccidia, and other forms, increase in number by multiple division. In addition to simple and multiple division, some protozoans exhibit more complicated reproductive phenomena that resemble sexual processes in higher animals.

The rapid multiplication of protozoans produces a severe invasion of the host. If the parasites live in the lumen, or cavity, of the digestive tract without penetrating the tissues proper, the host can usually cope successfully even with huge numbers, but if they penetrate the lining of the digestive tract, invade the blood, or are carried to various organs and tissues, serious consequences are likely to follow.

As already noted, some parasitic protozoans–including amoebae and some flagellates, ciliates, and some sporozoans–have but one host, infection resulting from the ingestion of food or water contaminated with the organisms eliminated with the droppings of infected animals.

In some such manner human beings acquire amoebae, which produce the disease known as amoebic dysentery, and various flagellates and ciliates that are responsible for digestive disturbances. Among the protozoan diseases of animals acquired in a similar manner are blackhead of chickens and turkeys, trichomoniasis of turkeys, and coccidiosis. Coccidiosis, often a serious disease of poultry, cattle, and sheep, is caused by coccidia, acquired as a result of swallowing feed or water that has become contaminated with the infective stages of the organisms.

There are various modifications of the general method of direct transmission just described. For instance, a breeding disease of cattle, known as bovine genital trichomoniasis, caused by flagellates known as trichomonads, is transmitted during copulation. Blackhead of turkeys and chickens may be transmitted not only by the birds' swallowing contaminated food or water but also through the ingestion of the eggs of poultry cecal worms (roundworm parasites of the ceca of chickens and turkeys) in which the infective organisms apparently become lodged.

As in the case of other parasites, certain protozoans are transmitted from host to host only through vectors. The vector-borne protozoan diseases are among the most serious and are very difficult to control. Malaria is transmitted by certain species of mosquitoes, which acquire the infection from the blood of an infected human being, and tick fever is transmitted by cattle ticks. Anaplasmosis, a protozoan disease of cattle related to tick fever, is also transmitted by ticks and by certain bloodsucking flies. Certain diseases of horses and other livestock in tropical countries are caused by trypanosomes, which are transmitted by insect vectors.

Worm Parasites

The worms parasitic in human beings, livestock, and poultry are visible to the naked eye in the adult stage, when their length ranges from a fraction of an inch to several feet. They are rather complex in structure, containing an alimentary canal (except tapeworms and thorny heads), excretory and nervous systems, highly complex reproductive systems, and other organs. The surface of the body has a hard covering which protects, the softer internal parts. Spines, hooks, teeth, and suckers are among the armatures of worms, these structures serving various purposes and enabling the parasites to attach themselves to the organs and tissues of the host. Worm parasites is the immature stages wander more or less extensively in the course of their invasion of a host, and some do so even as adults. They are provided with specialized contractile tissue or muscles for locomotion.

Parasitic worms multiply by a sexual process. Single individuals of some of these parasites contain both male and female reproductive systems; such forms are said to be bisexual, or hermaphroditic. In others, called unisexual, the males and females are separate individuals. In both cases the parasites develop from eggs.

Save for a few conspicuous exceptions, the eggs or the larvae that hatch from the eggs must leave the host animal in which they originate to undergo further development on the ground or elsewhere in the open or in intermediate hosts. Depending on the kinds of parasites concerned, susceptible hosts acquire worms by (1) swallowing infective eggs or larvae with feed or water, (2) the penetration of infective larvae through the skin, (3) swallowing intermediate hosts, as previously noted, and (4) being bitten by skin-piercing insects harbouring infective larvae. Slight or moderate infections in a host animal are increased in intensity by the entrance of additional infective organisms.

Worms occur in a variety of locations in the bodies of human beings and animals, the entire digestive tract, from the mouth to the large bowel, being one of the principal habitats of these pests. They also occur under the skin; in the muscles; in the abdominal cavity, liver, pancreas, spleen and kidneys; in the chest cavity, heart, and lungs; in connective tissue; in the brain and other parts of the central nervous system; in the eyes and other organs of sense; and in other locations. In fact, hardly an organ, tissue, or cavity in the human or animal body is absolutely resistant to invasion by worm parasites.

When worms get into the vital organs such as the liver, lungs, brain, or heart, they interfere with the proper functioning of these organs and do damage in other ways. The invasion of vital organs frequently results in more or less serious damage, the severity of the injuries and the resultant disability of the host being proportional, as a rule, to the number of invaders. It should not be assumed, however, that worms elsewhere in the body are comparatively harmless. On the contrary, some of the severest losses of sheep and cattle are due to stomach worms and related parasites living in the alimentary canal; they commonly attack the lining of the canal and often pierce the finer blood vessels of the stomach or intestinal wall, producing hemorrhage and injuring the host in other ways. The net result of such parasitism is anemia, emaciation, and death when the infection is heavy.

Although the worm parasites have much in common, they naturally fall into four distinct groups: (1) Flukes, or trematodes, (2) tapeworms, or cestodes, (3) roundworms, or nematodes, and (4) thorny heads, or acanthocephalids. These groups have more or less distinct habits and modes of transmission and will be considered separately.

Flukes

Flukes (Fig. 1), or trematodes, are soft, more or less flattened, usually leaflike parasitic worms. Some forms are more of less cylindrical, others are conical, and a few are elongated. These worms generally range in length and from a fraction of an inch up to about an inch or so, the largest known fluke attaining a length of 4 inches. Flukes are covered with minute spines and possess adhesive organs, in the form of muscular, cup-shaped suckers, that serve for attachment of the parasite to the tissues of the host. With the exception of one group, all flukes are bisexual.

The flukes that are of importance to human and animal health require snails as intermediate hosts. The mode of transmission is briefly as follows: The eggs of the parasites, eliminated as a rule with the host's droppings, hatch under favorable conditions of temperature and moisture. The larva penetrates into the body of a snail, within which it is considerably transformed in structure and where it produces one or more generations of very small flukes. The

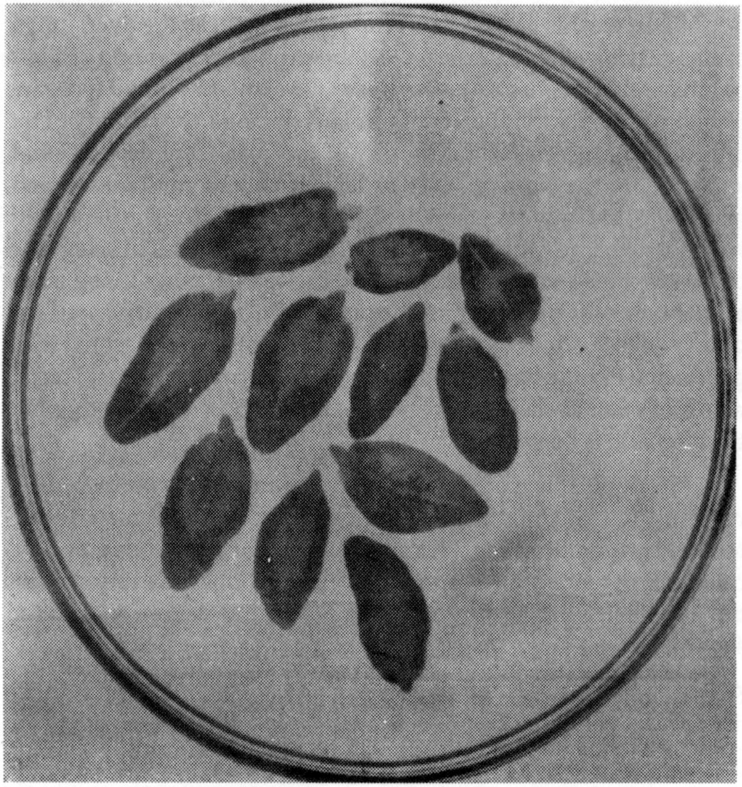

Fig. 1: Liver flukes of sheep, *Fasciola hepatica*.

stage that escapes from the snail is known as a cercaria, a single egg ultimately giving rise to many cercariae. The cercariae secrete a protective covering around themselves after they have lodged on vegetation, on the surface of water, or elsewhere. Grazing animals, such as cattle, sheep, swine, horses, and others, swallow the encysted cercariae with forage or water. The cercariae of some flukes penetrate the skin of the definitive host and thus bore into its body; others require a second intermediate host. The cercariae of lung flukes of swine penetrate into crayfishes, and hogs become infected by swallowing the parasitized crayfishes.

Flukes are known to produce serious diseases in man and animals in various parts of the world, but fortunately some of the most harmful do not occur in this country. The only flukes that are definitely known to be important in the United States are the liver flukes that commonly parasitize cattle, sheep, and goats and may also occur from time to time in horses, swine, and other animals. These flukes produce injury as a result of their migrations in the body and in other ways. The activities of the flukes produce extensive destruction of the liver tissue, and more or less extensive hemorrhage may result from the rupture of blood vessels.

Tapeworms

Like the flukes, all tapeworms are strictly parasitic. Tapeworms of economic importance occur as adults in the intestine and as bladder worms in various locations outside the alimentary canal, including the muscles, abdominal cavity, liver, lungs, brain, eye, and other organs and tissues. On casual inspection there appears to be little resemblance between a bladder worm and an adult tapeworm. The fact is, however, that bladder worms are the larval stages of intestinal tapeworms. The head of the bladder worm resembles that of the adult tapeworm in practically all respects. Bladder worms vary considerably in size, some being only about half an inch or less in diameter, whereas others are much larger. The so-called hydatids that parasitize man as well as cattle, sheep, swine, and other animals may attain the size of a child's head.

Adult tapeworms range in length from a fraction of an inch to several feet. They are elongated, flattened worms, each individual consisting of a head, an unsegmented neck, and a chain of segments. The head is provided with four suckers or similar organs of attachment and in many cases with hooks also. The neck is more or less constricted, and the segments behind the neck vary considerably in shape in different species. Those immediately below the neck are the immature segments, and the mature ones, each containing both male and female reproductive organs, are farther down in the chain. The segments toward the end of the chain are known as the ripe, gravid, segments, and each contains hundreds of eggs. The gravid segments of some tapeworms become detached either singly or in groups and pass out of the body with the excreta; in others detachment does not take place, the tapeworm eggs being liberated into the host's intestine and excreted. In either case the eggs serve as the starting point for new infections, the intermediate host swallowing them in contaminated feed or water.

Various animals serve as intermediate hosts. The tapeworms affecting cattle, sheep, and goats develop in small free-living mites that live on grass; those affecting chickens develop in various beetles and other insects and in other invertebrates; some of those affecting dogs develop in rabbits, some in sheep, cattle, goats, and swine, and some in lice and fleas. Of the tapeworms affecting man, one species develops in swine, another in cattle (Fig. 2), and one in certain freshwater fishes. The definitive host becomes infected as a result of swallowing the intermediate host in whole or in part.

Since worm parasites that live in cavities of the body have less opportunity for doing serious damage than those that occur in or have intimate contact with tissues, it is obvious that bladder worms, which as a rule occur in tissues, produce more injury than the corresponding adult tapeworms. Furthermore, bladder worms occurring in the liver, lungs, brain, eyes, and other organs produce more injury than those that occur in the abdominal cavity attached to the mesenteries. Bladder worms that get into the brain are particularly dangerous, a disease of sheep known as gid being caused by the presence in the brain of a bladder worm an inch or so in diameter. Man sometimes harbours the bladder worm or the pork tapeworm, these cystic worms in man showing a predilection for the brain and eye. Hydatids, already mentioned, occur in man as well as in animals, becoming localized principally in the liver and lungs. Because of their size and location, they produce serious disturbances. Infection in man requires surgical intervention. Though adult tapeworms in the intestine produce more or less injury

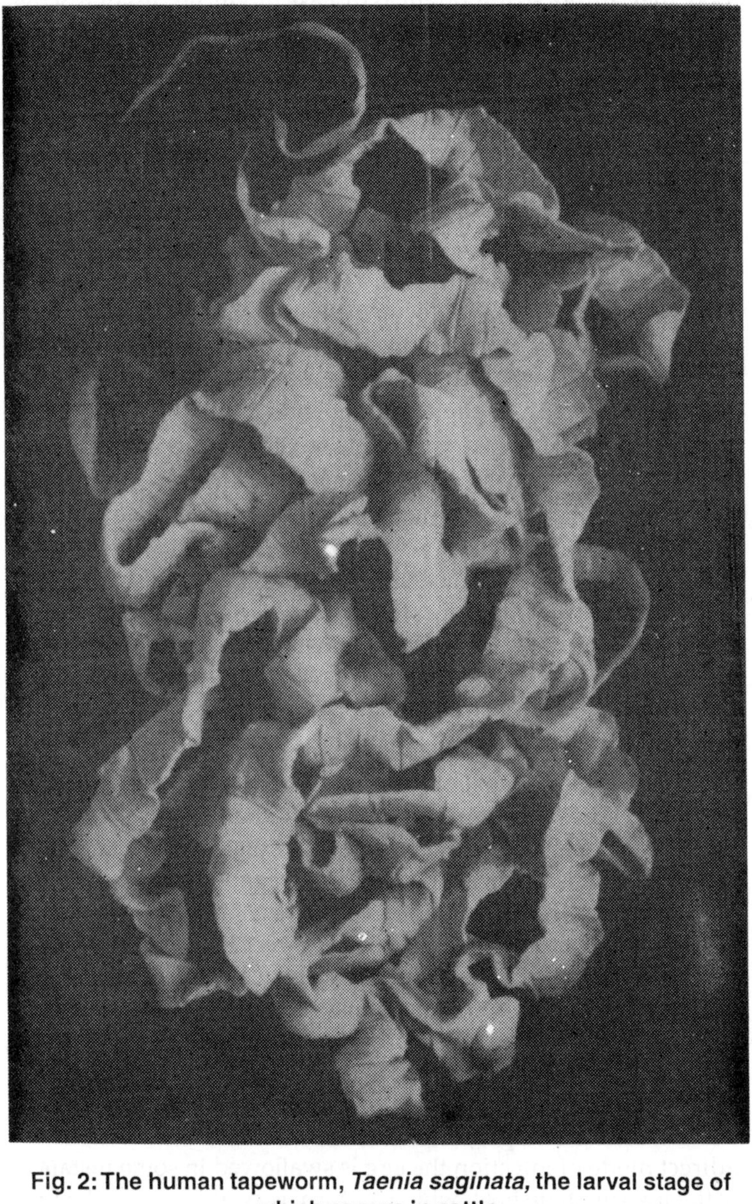

Fig. 2: The human tapeworm, *Taenia saginata,* the larval stage of which occurs in cattle.

to the intestinal lining, irritate its nerve endings, and rob the host of food, they are not so important as disease producers, in spite of their relatively large size, as adult flukes and roundworms.

Roundworms

Roundworms, or nematodes, constitute a group of rather slender cylindrical worms, more or less attenuated at both ends. Some nematodes are free-living, some parasitize plants, and others are parasitic in man and animals. The last-named group shows a wide range in size, the smallest ones being but a fraction of an inch long and as thin as a fine silk thread. The large ones attain a length of about a foot and are as thick as or thicker than an ordinary lead pencil. The kidney worm of dogs, which occurs in the abdominal cavity as well as in the kidneys, is the largest known nematode and may attain a length of about 3½ feet and a width of about half an inch.

Nematodes occur in a variety of locations in and outside of the alimentary canal, some of them wandering extensively as larvae and as adults, thereby getting into situations from which, sometimes, they cannot extricate themselves and in which they ultimately die. Their presence in strange locations produces injury by pressure on tissues and in other ways. All organs and tissues of the human body previously mentioned as habitats of parasites, and others as well, are subject to attack by nematodes.

As a rule, parasitic nematodes occur as male and female worms. Usually the eggs are expelled by the female worm into the alimentary canal or cavities that communicate with it and reach the outside with the excreta. The eggs of nematodes that live in the urinary system are discharged with the urine. The eggs of species that require intermediate hosts are usually infective when they reach the outside, whereas those of species that have a direct life history undergo development before they can infect new hosts. The infective, unhatched eggs of the large intestinal roundworms, or ascarids, of pigs and those of some other forms are swallowed by the host and hatch within it. The eggs of the sheep stomach worm and related parasites hatch on the ground, where the larvae undergo considerable development before they become infective. In the indirect mode of infection the egg is swallowed in some instances by the intermediate host, which, in turn, is swallowed by the final host, which thus becomes infected. For example, hogs acquire longworms by eating earthworms that harbour them in the infective stage, the earthworms having acquired the lungworm larvae by swallowing lungworm eggs with swine manure. In other indirect modes of transmission, the eggs hatch within the nematode, and the larvae get into the host's blood, transmission to another host being effected through skin-piercing insects, particularly flies and mosquitoes, which act as intermediate hosts. Heart worms of dogs and related filarid nematodes of man and animals are transmitted in this manner. Other methods of transmission also occur and are discussed in the various articles dealing with specific nematode infections.

Nematodes are among the most injurious parasites of man, domestic animals, and poultry. They cause trichinosis, a disease of the muscles of man and swine; hookworm disease in man and animals, characterized by anemia, stunting, and emaciation; stomach worm disease in cattle, sheep, and goat and strongylidosis in horses, which are characterized by similar symptoms; heart worm disease in dogs and a more or less related disease known as filariasis in man and animals; verminous bronchitis and pneumonia in all food animals; nodular disease in sheep; gapeworm disease in chickens and turkeys; and many other serious conditions. The anemia characteristic of some of these diseases is produced by the bloodsucking activities of the parasites and leads to malnutrition and wasting; the invasion of the lungs by lungworms and wandering larvae of other nematodes produces the bronchitis and pneumonia characteristic of other diseases; the lodgement of worms in the heart and principal blood vessels produces profound disturbances in circulation and respiration; the invasion of the muscles produces severe pain; and other activities of nematodes produce either acute disease or a gradual undermining of the host's vitality.

Thorny Heads

Thorny heads, or acanthocephalids, constitute a group of elongated cylindrical worms related to the nematodes but differing from them in a number of ways, especially in the presence of an alimentary canal. The name "thorny heads" is derived from the peculiar anatomical structure characteristic of these worms, namely, a retractile proboscis, or snout, armed with hooks. The sexes are separate, and the life history is indirect. Only one species, the thorny head of swine, is of importance to the livestock industry.

Intermediate Hosts and Vectors

As already stated, some parasites are transmitted from one host animal to another directly, without the intervention of intermediate hosts. Intermediate hosts play an essential role in the transmission of others, however. When more than one intermediate host is involved, the one which the parasite invades first is called the first intermediate host and the next the second intermediate host. In this article the term "intermediate host" is restricted to animals that harbour the larval stages of worm parasites. Hosts that transmit the minute unicellular organisms known as protozoa are referred to as vectors (carriers). Knowledge of intermediate hosts and vectors is as important as knowledge of the parasites they harbour. Control of parasites that require intermediate hosts or vectors frequently requires as much or more attention to the latter as to the parasites themselves. Without mosquitoes, for example, there would be no malaria. Tick or splenetic fever, which at one time was widespread in cattle in the South, has almost completely disappeared as a result of a systematic campaign of tick eradication.

Common intermediate hosts and vectors of parasites are ticks, flies, mosquitoes, beetles, snails, slugs, and other small invertebrate animals that are usually common in farm lots, barnyards, and pastures. Larger animals also may serve as intermediate hosts. In fact, almost any animal, including domestic animals and human beings, may serve as an intermediate host of parasites.

Ticks and biting insects, particularly flies and mosquitoes, are especially adapted to serve as intermediate hosts or vectors of parasites that occur in the blood. Malaria in man, tick fever and anaplasmosis in cattle, heart worm infection in dogs, and other parasitic diseases are transmitted by bloodsucking insects and related forms. Dung beetles, snails, slugs, earthworms, and other small creatures that feed on animal manure serve as intermediate hosts for specific parasites. These hosts ingest, or swallow, parasite eggs and larvae present in manure, and the definitive host becomes infected by eating the parasitised intermediate host. In other cases parasites are acquired by animals and human beings by eating the flesh and other tissues of parasitized animals. For instance, dogs acquire certain tapeworms by eating rabbits that harbour bladder worms, the immature stages of these pests. Man acquires certain tapeworms by eating raw or rare beef or pork infected with bladder worms, and he acquires trichinosis by eating raw or rare trichina-infected pork.

Poisonous Plants as Causes of Disease

Poisonous plants occupy an important place among the causes of animal diseases. Owing to their wide distribution and relative abundance, such plants have been responsible for heavy livestock losses in many sections of the country. The action of poisonous plants on animals varies greatly. It is dependent not only on the character and amount of toxic substance present, but also on the animals involved, since the same plant may be much more toxic to certain species of animals than to others. Often there is considerable variation in toxicity in the different parts of a plant and at different stages of its growth, and there may be some difference in the toxicity of the same species of plants growing in different localities and environments.

Poisoning may result from a single feeding or from repeated feedings scattered over a period of days or weeks. Many poisonous plants can be eaten daily in relatively small amounts over a long period of time with no apparent injury, whereas others eaten in the same way may produce a cumulative effect, the animals eventually developing acute symptoms of poisoning some time after they have stopped eating the plant.,

Chemical analyses of plants proved to be poisonous have resulted in many cases in the isolation of the specific principles responsible for the trouble. Since there are many different toxic substances in poisonous plants, the diseases resulting from their consumption show a wide variation in the symptoms observed and the tissue changes that may occur. Certain species of plants may produce their primary effects on specific tissues or organs of the body, such as the nervous system, digestive tract, liver, or kidneys, causing manifestations that may easily be mistaken for diseases originating from other causes.

The duration of the diseases caused by poisonous plants varies from the acute, rapidly fatal condition produced by highly toxic substances to chronic cases resulting from the cumulative action of some of the slower acting poisons.

In addition to those poisonous plants in which the toxic principles are normal constituents and more or less uniform in all plants of the same species, other plants, ordinarily considered nontoxic, when grown on certain soils may become poisonous owing to the presence in the soil of the very poisonous element selenium. The presence of selenium in the soil, combined with the ability of certain plants, which may include native species as well as some cultivated ones, to assimilate this element in sufficient quantities to render them toxic to animals, has created an unusual disease problem which in some areas has resulted in considerable livestock loss.

Nutritional Deficiencies as Causes of Disease

As dramatic as the researches of Pasteur, Lister, Koch, and the others who firmly established the germ theory of disease has been the discovery that errors in diet can cause specific diseases and other debilitating conditions in animals and man no less extreme than those due to germs and other organisms. In fact, it is now recognised that certain animal diseases may be caused by the combined effects of nutritional deficiencies or excesses and of infection. In some instances the dietary deficiency precedes the invasion of the body by organisms, while in others an infectious disease, once established in a well-nourished animal, may lead to nutritional complications if the functions of digestion and assimilation of food or the excretion of waste products are disturbed.

It is now recognized that the maintenance of life and health in animals depends on the orderly coordination of numerous chemical and physical reactions within the body cells and fluids. Some of these reactions are concerned with the transformation of food into heat to maintain body temperature and energy for body activities, and others with the synthesis of building materials to be used in growth, in repair or replacement of essential constituents of body tissues and fluids, or in such functions as reproduction. Some components of food appear to act merely as catalysts, starting or helping along these complex reactions. These substances are probably used up in the process and apparently do not remain as definite structural elements.

Whenever a vital function or series of vital reactions is interrupted owing to continued failure of the diet to supply sufficient quantities of essential nutrients or to the inability of the body to utilize these nutrients because of a dietary imbalance, the so-called nutritional diseases develop. Toxic manifestations can also result from the feeding of an excess of some nutrients. The symptoms of these diseases depend on the particular functions of the body that are affected. Some nutritional deficiencies inhibit the growth of animals; in others growth continues, but faulty development occurs. Detection of the early symptoms of nutritional diseases and an understanding of the pathological and biochemical changes involved are proving to be of great value in diagnosing diseases of nutritional origin and thereby making it possible to work out means for their control.

The recognition of the essential nature of such dietary factors as certain minerals, vitamins, and amino acids, along with protein in general, carbohydrates, fats, and water, has led to the conception of a complete or balanced diet. Such a diet, however, must vary with the food requirements of animals according to species, age, rate of growth, sex, and amount of physical work as well as with such functions as reproduction and lactation. Recent developments that have led to outstanding advances in the field of animal nutrition have included the isolation and synthesis of practically all of the known vitamins, recognition of the need for several minerals in very small amounts, the demonstration of the essential nature of several amino acids, and a better understanding of how to preserve nutritive values in harvested crops. It is now evident that many diseases which were formerly believed to be caused by some obscure infection or some toxic principle in the feed are really due to a deficiency of essential nutritive factors.

At the time this book went to press, the drugs and other materials mentioned in various articles–chiefly as disinfectants, insecticides, and anthelmintics–were still available for veterinary and medical use. Under war conditions, however, it is possible that some of these materials may become scarce or unavailable. In that case, the reader should obtain professional advice from the Department of Agriculture, the State experiment station, a local veterinarian, or the county agent as to available substitutes.

Chapter 3

PROTECTIVE MECHANISMS AGAINST DISEASE

Adolph Eichhorn, Merritt P. Sarles & N.R. Ellis[1]

[1] *Adolph Eichhorn is Director of the Animal Disease Station; Merritt P. Sarles is Assistant Parasitologist, Zoological Division; and N.R. Ellis is Senior Chemist, Animal Nutrition Division, Bureau of Animal Industry. Dr. Eichhorn prepared portions of the text relating to bacterial and virus diseases; Dr. Sarles contributed the section on parasitic diseases; and Mr. Ellis prepared the section on nutrition and disease resistance.*

Probably the most brilliant achievement of modern medical science has been the gradual disclosure of nature's methods of producing immunity against disease, and the use of these methods to protect human beings and animals by artificial immunization. Not only livestock producers but everyone should understand the fundamentals of this process.

Bacterial and Virus Diseases

In the prevention and treatment of diseases of animals a knowledge of the principles of immunity is highly desirable, especially when biological products, such as vaccines, bacterins, toxoids, and immune serum, are to be used.

In its true sense immunity denotes complete resistance to a disease, but since all individuals of a species can seldom be made resistant enough to withstand severe exposure, the term is now used chiefly in a relative sense; that is, it does not necessarily mean absolute resistance, but signifies that the natural resistance, if any, of an individual has been increased to a certain degree, which may be slight or marked, usually the latter. Susceptibility is the opposite of resistance, denoting that an animal of a certain species or the large majority of animals in a given species may contract a disease readily if exposed to it.

Natural and Acquired Immunity

Immunity may be natural or acquired. Natural immunity to a specific disease is inherited, and the degree of immunity varies considerably in different individuals. Just as no two animals are exactly alike in physical appearance and mental attributes, no two are exactly alike in susceptibility or resistance to disease. When a herd of swine has been exposed to hog cholera, for example, a few animals commonly die within 48 to 72 hours after the first symptoms develop; others–probably the majority–are sick for 4 to 10 days before dying; some recover after being slightly sick, and some after being very sick; and a few may show no indication of illness. The last group would be considered naturally immune.

Again, horses and cattle may be exposed directly to hog cholera, but they never contract this disease. Such natural resistance is known as species immunity, meaning that all or most individuals of a species of animals are resistant or immune to a specific disease.

Other factors operate in resistance to a disease, chief of which are the severity of exposure and the virulence of the germs or virus causing the disease. It can be readily understood, therefore, that resistance is a complex problem and that natural immunity may be broken down in many instances by severe exposure.

For an understanding of acquired immunity it is necessary first to be familiar with certain physiological processes.

The inroads of bacteria, parasites, and other foreign substances into the body of a susceptible animal stimulate three remarkable, complex, and somewhat related protective reactions: Inflammation, immunization, and repair. By means of these processes the body attempts to localize, neutralize, and ultimately destroy the foreign organisms or substances; to produce chemical substances–antibodies–antagonistic to or protective against the foreign materials; and to repair and compensate for injuries sustained.

Two types of physiological elements, namely, cells and antibodies, are chiefly concerned in these processes. Of primary importance, since they produce the antibodies, are the living, microscopic cells of which all tissues are composed, and especially those of the blood and connective tissues, including the specialized larger phagocytic, or devouring, cells called macrophages. Macrophages are present in all the connective or supporting tissues of the body and are concentrated in great numbers in the liver, spleen, and lymph nodes. The cells of this protective system are of great importance against infection, since they not only take up and devour foreign organisms and substances but also appear to be the main elements concerned in the production of antibodies.

Thus an animal's body may be considered a battleground in which the invading forces seek to overcome the defenses. The aim of the livestock owner and his ally, the veterinarian, is to aid animals in acquiring sufficient immunity to resist the invading organisms.

Active and Passive Immunity

Acquired resistance can be increased by one or a combination of several means. If the animal produces its own antibodies, the resultant immunity is called active immunity. If the resistance of an animal is increased by the injection of antibodies produced by another animal, the immunity is known as passive.

Animals acquire an active immunity to certain diseases when they have survived a natural or modified course of the disease produced either by infection with the particular germs or by inoculation with their specific vaccines, bacterins, or toxins. In these cases, the animal produces its own immunity, either because it had the disease naturally or because it sustained a less severe form of infection produced intentionally by artificial means. Intentional active immunization is commonly called vaccination, although the latter term, to be exact, signifies that a vaccine has been used to produce the protection.

Passive immunity is produced in an animal by the introduction of immunizing substances obtained from an actively immune animal. Such immunity is usually conferred by the injection of blood serum from immunized animals; such serum carries with it the substances by which the protection is conferred. The immunizing substances (antibodies) of an actively immunized animal are known also as immune bodies. In relation to infectious diseases, they comprise two classes. Those acting on bacteria are antibacterial, as, for instance, anti-white-scours serum and anti anthrax serum, whereas those acting on toxins are called antitoxin, as, for instance, tetanus antitoxin.

Active immunity develops only after 1 or 2 weeks, whereas passive immunity is established immediately after the injection. Passive immunity does not protect animals for a long period; it usually disappears within 3 to 6 weeks. This is due to the fact that as soon as the injected immune bodies are eliminated from the animal organism, the immunity is ended. In active immunity, however, the stimulation of the infection on the body cells causes the prolonged development of immune bodies, and thus a more lasting immunity is produced.

It can be seen from this brief description that active immunity has a great advantage over passive immunity, and the tendency is to produce active immunity whenever possible. On the other hand, there are times when it becomes necessary to employ means by which the spread of a disease can be immediately checked, and in such instances passive immunity has the advantage, since it affords immediate protection against infection; in some instances it also exerts a curative action. Frequently, both methods are used in a combined inoculation by which the animal is given immediate and also lasting protection against an infectious disease. This form of immunization is known as the simultaneous method, a familiar example of which is virus-serum inoculation against hog cholera.

Scientists the world over have expended much effort in attempts to discover and perfect effective and at the same time practical means of immunizing animals against the more destructive of the infectious diseases. Large sums have been appropriated for the advancement of these researches, both from governmental sources and by private gifts and endowments. The goal sought is the discovery of some means by which immunity may be conveyed to a large number of animals at the least expense. After successful vaccination, the animal is sufficiently protected to withstand exposure that would have proved deadly before vaccination was performed. The same principle is used in protecting man from many diseases; for example, smallpox and diphtheria.

It appears natural, then, that the best and surest results from immunization should be expected in those diseases in which the specific cause has been definitely established and for which means of effective protection are known. This is the case in actual practice.

Vaccination

In localities where a disease appears year after year it is advisable to vaccinate susceptible animals while they are healthy; that is, before exposure. It is not advisable to delay the immunization until the disease actually makes its appearance. Such a practice may prove costly because of the time required before actual protection is established and also because some of the animals may already have become infected though not yet showing symptoms.

The object of vaccination, as already noted, is to induce in the animal a reaction, sometimes a mild form of the disease, which stimulates the body to develop antibodies against the infective agent. It is very important that the vaccination be undertaken when the animal is in a healthy condition, as any devitalization will adversely affect the immunization. It is well known that the presence of the infection is not the sole cause of a diseased condition. In most cases the combined effects of various contributing factors are necessary. Immediately after the invasion of the infective agent, the protective mechanism of the body is set in motion, and the disease results only if the attack is stronger than the defence; that is, if the animal is not capable of producing sufficient antibodies.

Influences that tend to weaken the normal functioning of the body include overwork, exposure to cold, lack of proper feed, and shipment of animals over long distances, especially in stormy weather. Chronic infections also may lower resistance. In particular, a disease condition or a parasitic infestation may predispose an animal to infection, because while it is still fighting one disease it is called upon to combat a new invader. The failure under such circumstances explains the frequent occurrence of two diseases simultaneously, or of one following immediately after another. A disease devitalizes the body and prepares it for an attack by either latent or invading germs of a secondary infection. This situation is often observed in hog cholera, equine influenza, canine distemper, and other maladies. The formation of antibodies is influenced also by the age of the animal; neither very young nor old animals respond to vaccination so well as those between these extremes.

Susceptibility to disease is also influenced to some extent by breeding practices, such as inbreeding, as well as by selection for high productivity or performance. (See the article The Relation of Genetics to Disease.) Feeding, discussed later, also plays an important part.

To increase the chances of success in vaccination, therefore, it is advisable to eliminate all debilitating influences before the immunization is carried out. In vaccinating against hog cholera or canine distemper, for instance, the animals should be freed of parasites if any are present and should be protected from exposure to cold and dampness. Any vitamin or mineral deficiency in the diet should also be corrected. It is a mistake to depend solely on vaccination; every effort should be made to eliminate all adverse conditions that might interfere with its success.

Preparations Used in Producing Immunity

For the production of immunity to various kinds of infection, veterinary research has developed numerous biological products. The preparation and distribution of these biologics in pure and potent form contribute greatly to the safety of modern livestock production. Probably the most familiar class of biologics is the vaccines.

A vaccine is an attenuated, weakened, or even apparently dead virus of the disease, specially prepared so that it will perform its function with the least possible danger to the animal. The reduction of virulence is accomplished by subjecting the virus to heat, desiccation (drying), or other unfavourable influences strong enough to weaken but not to destroy it. Examples are anthrax vaccine and blackleg vaccine. In some instances an organism modified in virulence is used for immunizing purposes, as, for instance, in bovine brucellosis (Bang's disease); or, again, an unattenuated virus may be used when it has passed through certain species of animals, a procedure that increases its virulence for that particular species but reduces it for other species. For instance, suspensions of a brain emulsion of fixed rabies virus passed through rabbits are used for immunizing other species of animals against rabies. In the use of viruses for immunizing purposes, the general opinion formerly was that immunization with "killed" virus had not been successful. Recently, however, very dependable immunity has been produced with such virus, as illustrated by successful immunization against equine encephalomyelitis with chick-embryo vaccine, in the preparation of which the virus is killed (Fig. 1). The vaccine has proved highly effective not only in experimental tests but also in extensive field use.

Bacterins, another class of biologics, are standardized suspensions of killed pathogenic bacteria and their products in physiological salt solution[2] or in oil. Immunization with bacterins against certain diseases, such as hemorrhagic septicemia, blackleg, and other infections, is now an established procedure. Bacterins are standardized to a definite number of dead organisms per cubic centimeter. This procedure involves either the counting of stained organisms in a special counting chamber or the use of a photoelectric

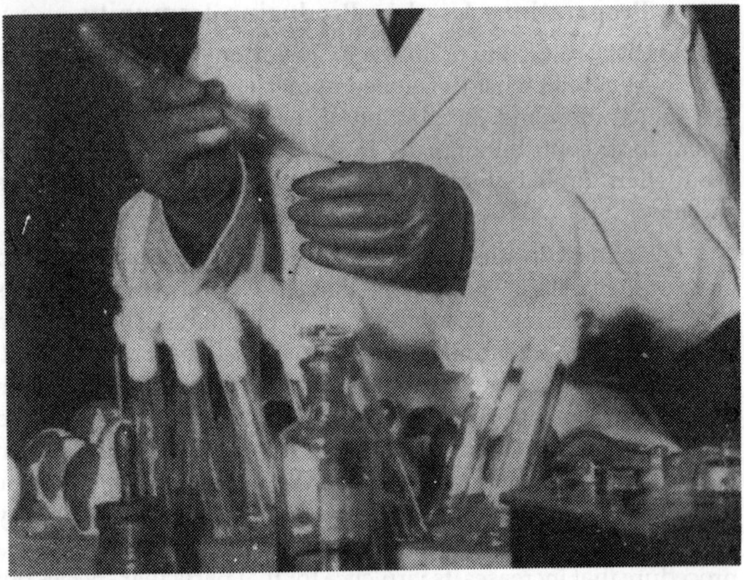

Fig. 1: A step in the production of chick-embryo vaccine, used for protecting horses against equine encephalomyelitis. The use of chick embryos as a culture medium is one of the newer developments in the preparation of veterinary biologics.

---

[2] This term signifies approximately the same dilution of salt (sodium chloride) that is found in body fluids, usually 0.85 percent.

apparatus which determines the density of a suspension by measuring the quantity of light refracted or absorbed in passing through the suspension. The latter method has greatly simplified the standardization of such suspensions.

Another biological product used in combating disease is immune blood serum (or immune serum), so-called because of its content of immunizing bodies. When injected into the body, such serum, by reason of the protective nature of the antibodies, does one of two things. It either exerts an inhibitory (stopping) action against the virulent virus or acts as an antitoxin, neutralizing the poisonous products (toxins) of the disease-producing organisms.

For the preparation of immune serum, horses are generally used, principally because their size makes possible the drawing of large volumes of blood. In treating a horse for the production of antitoxin, small quantities of the respective toxin are first injected, for the production of antibacterial serum, suspensions of the bacteria of the specific disease are injected. Periodical tests are made of the potency of the serum, to determine among other things its ability to protect other animals. When a suitable potency is obtained, a quantity of blood is drawn from the jugular vein into sterile containers. After standing 24 hours, the separated serum is siphoned off, properly preserved, filtered if necessary, and put into final containers.

Immune serum is assimilated most rapidly if administered intravenously (into the veins), especially if therapeutic (healing or curative) action is desired. For prophylactic (preventive) purposes, the injection is made either intramuscularly (into the muscles) or subcutaneously (under the skin).

Toxoids (anatoxins), consisting of detoxified disease-producing toxins, are gaining in importance and are used very extensively for immunization purposes; examples are diphtheria toxoid and tetanus toxoid.

Other products employed for the protection of animals against disease are sensitized vaccines, sensitized bacterins, germ-free extracts, natural and artificial aggressions, and bacterial filtrates. Although the methods of preparation and characteristics of these biologics vary somewhat, the principle of action is essentially the same. It consists in the production of protective substances against corresponding infections.

In the course of their studies bacteriologists propagate bacteria on various kinds of culture media and sometimes produce different strains, comparable to the various strains of plants and animals (Fig. 2). For the purpose of immunization, vaccines or bacterins are sometimes prepared from a single strain of an organism, constituting what is called a monovalent vaccine or bacterin. When prepared from two or more strains, the product is known as polyvalent. A polyvalent vaccine or bacterin is not the same as a, "mixed" vaccine, or "mixed" bacterin, which is a mixture of different kinds of bacteria.

At times an autogenous (self-generated) vaccine is employed–that is, one prepared for an organism isolated from an animal affected with a disease and used for the protection of the same animal or similar animals in the locality. An autogenous vaccine has the

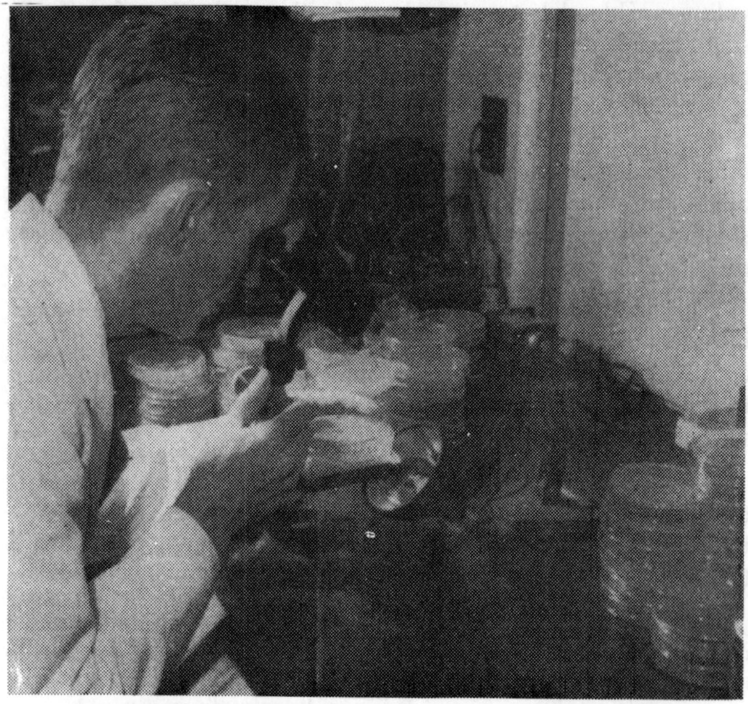

Fig. 2: Examining cultures of *Brucella* organisms at the Animal Disease Station of the Bureau of Animal Industry. Most of the experimental work leading to successful vaccination against brucellosis by means of a selected strain of the organism was conducted here.

advantage of containing the particular strain of organism that caused the infection.

Although one injection of the vaccine or bacterin induces the production of antibodies, naturally repeated injections produce a higher degree of resistance, which often is hastened by successively larger doses. The correct quantities are established through experimentation.

Biological Products as Diagnostic Agents

A highly useful specialized class of biological products is that comprising diagnostic agents. As the name signifies, these are used not for preventing or curing a disease, but rather for indicating its presence. The diagnostic agent tuberculin, used in detecting tuberculosis in cattle, swine, and poultry, is a familiar example.

There are three principal methods of tuberculin testing–the intradermic, subcutaneous, and ophthalmic, of which the first is the method now principally used. It consists in the injection of tuberculin into the dermis, the true skin. If the animal is tuberculous, a characteristic swelling later occurs at the site of injection. Expert knowledge of the technique of the test is necessary for its proper use and for interpretation of the results.

The accuracy, as diagnostic agents, of tuberculin and of mallein (used to detect glanders in horses) is so great that veterinary officials destroy reacting animals even though they appear healthy. The animals are slaughtered with absolute confidence that in the great majority of instances the post mortem examination will justify the diagnosis, made solely on the findings of the biological test.

Ability to detect latent cases and to verify clinical ones is a valuable aid in eradication measures. Early diagnosis of such diseases also obviates the necessity of long periods of quarantine. For combating dourine in horses the complement-fixation method of diagnosis has given excellent results. This is also the laboratory test used for the diagnosis of glanders; the mallein test–comparable in principle to the tuberculin test-is used chiefly in testing for glanders on farms.

The complement-fixation method (*12*)[3] is based on the phenomenon of hemolysis, or the dissolution of red blood cells. When

[3] Italic numbers in parentheses refer to Literature Cited.

the cells dissolve, the hemoglobin in them is set free in the surrounding fluid. Research has shown that when the red blood cells of an animal are introduced into another animal of a different species, the latter's blood acquires the ability to dissolve the blood cells of the first animal. The dissolving action is due to the development of antibodies that acquire the power described; and the reaction–hemolysis–takes place readily in laboratory equipment, such as a glass container. The acquired so-called hemolytic property of the blood depends on two substances, one of which, the hemolysin, has been found to resist heating to about 56°-58°C., whereas the other, the complement, is rendered inactive by this degree of heating. When the complement is "fixed" by union with a specific substance in the serum of the animal under test (the substance resulting from the presence of the disease), the red corpuscles are not dissolved but settle to the bottom of the test tube. This represents a positive reaction, indicating disease. In the case of a healthy animal, no fixation of complement occurs; consequently hemolysis takes place, and the test is read as negative. The Wassermann test for syphilis, widely used in human medicine, is a complement-fixation test.

Still other diagnostic tests that have been extensively applied in recent years are the agglutination test for the detection of brucellosis in cattle (*7*) and the rapid whole-blood test for pullorum disease in chickens (*5*). In testing for brucellosis, use is made of the production by the body of specific antibodies, previously mentioned, that are believed to assist the animal in resisting the disease. One of these substances, existing in the body of an animal infected with brucellosis, is known as agglutinin. It is present in the blood serum in a quantity that depends on the extent and activity of the infection. When serum from an infected animal is brought into contact with a preparation of *Brucella* organisms, called antigen, the organisms gather together in clumps and are technically described as agglutinated. This principle is the basis of the agglutination test, which has been found to compare favourably in accuracy with the tuberculin test for tuberculosis. There are two methods of making the agglutination test, one of which involves the use of a tube and the other a plate. The choice depends somewhat on conditions favourable to the use of each. In general they are equally efficient.

In the control of pullorum disease in poultry, which for many years caused extensive losses, the principle of agglutination is likewise employed. The form of test principally used is the rapid whole-blood test, the basis of which is a stained antigen. The discovery through research that a chemical stain added to antigen makes the reaction more easily seen has greatly facilitated the detection of pullorum disease in poultry. With modern equipment for holding and testing the birds, the rate of handling them is very rapid, usually less then 2 minutes each.

Diagnostics are prepared and used in various ways, and the reactions of animals to them are likewise widely different, requiring, specialized training for their proper application and for correct interpretation of the results.

Biological Products Not to be Used As Sole Reliance

The remarkable results often obtained with biological products in combating disease have unfortunately led to a tendency to rely on them solely. A much better course is to give due consideration to the various factors associated with the condition concerned and utilize all measures that will contribute to the desired result. Thus, in treating a case of fistulous withers, it is not enough merely to inject a polyvalent vaccine and then wait for the animal to get well. Supportive treatment, including the possible aid of surgery, should also be considered.

Further, in attempting to control a disease, it is not sufficient to limit activities to vaccination of the exposed and susceptible animals; it is equally essential to inaugurate the necessary sanitary measures, and if possible the source of infection should be looked for and eliminated.

Animals suffering from infectious diseases may be thought of as living factories that produce and distribute vast numbers of disease germs. Thus they are more or less directly a menace to others, and the healthy animals should be segregated from the sick. This is best accomplished by removing the healthy animals immediately to a disease-free environment. In some cases destruction of the infected animals is the wisest course. Thorough disinfection (see Disinfection and Disinfectants) and efforts to minimize the danger of exposure to possible subsequent infection should also be a part of the disease-control plan.

As already indicated, the passive form of immunity, conferred on animals as an immediate protective measure, is of short duration, lasting at times not more than a month. Therefore, when the danger of infection is still believed to exist, steps must be taken to guard against losses when the temporary immunity expires. In such instances the passive immunization should be followed with the active form, which renders the animal safe for a much longer time.

Importance of Proper Administration and Care of Biologics

The technique of administration must be given careful attention if best results are to be obtained. The animal to be treated should be properly prepared; the site of inoculation should be carefully cleansed and disinfected; and all instruments and utensils coming in contact with the product to be administered should be thoroughly sterilized. Bacterial suspensions should be shaken vigourously to insure an even mixture, and great care should be taken to see that the dose administered is accurate. When dealing with such products as anthrax vaccine and hog cholera virus, it is important that the empty containers and unused portions of such products be disposed of properly. If they should be carelessly thrown aside, there is a possibility that they might be a factor in causing future outbreaks of the disease. It is always essential that the products intended for use in vaccinating should be pure, potent, and used with proper skill. In accordance with the provisions of the Virus-Serum-Toxin Act, a Federal statute, most biological products for the prevention and cure of infections in animals are prepared under license of the United States Department of Agriculture. The products should preferably be administered by a trained veterinarian.

Most biological products are sensitive to light and heat, and directions for their proper storage should be strictly followed to prevent deterioration. Practitioners have no ready means of recognizing changes that may have taken place in a product. If its previous handling or storage has been faulty, a biologic may have become inert. This phase of biological treatment is especially important in connection with highly infectious diseases. When an inert vaccine is used in such cases, both the veterinarian and the stock owner are often unable to explain the subsequent appearance of the disease. Unfortunately, such cases are rather numerous, and from the writer's personal experience in testing vaccines from various sources he can state that the failure to keep the vaccines under proper conditions is responsible for many such disappointing results. The importance of using dependable biologics and having them properly stored and competently administered can scarcely be overemphasized.

Although many different products are prepared for the prevention and treatment of disease, some stand out prominently over others in their specific action and rank among the triumphs of modern medicine. Diphtheria antitoxin, tetanus antitoxin, rabies vaccine, anthrax vaccine, blackleg aggressin, and calf scours serum have given results absolutely unattainable by any other means. Yet it must be remembered that a biological remedy is not specific in the sense that it will always prevent or cure. Neither do the diagnostic agents always detect disease. To the trained mind, these limitations are not unexpected; they exist because the ever-varying individual factor is involved.

Each year of research and experience extends the usefulness of biologic therapeutics. Increasing knowledge also continues to emphasize these basic points: (1) Biologic remedies should be used early, in full dosage; (2) they must be potent at the time of use; (3) antisepsis must be thorough; and (4) supplementary treatment that tends to ameliorate symptoms or conserve vital powers is a valuable adjunct to the use of biologics.

Protective Mechanisms Against Parasites

Until a few years ago it was considered improbable that there is any protective mechanism of immunity against animal parasites. The few reactions observed in parasitic infections were believed to by fundamentally different from those in other types of infection. It is now well established, however, that many animals do manifest both natural and acquired protective mechanisms against parasites and that these are basically similar to those observed in virus and bacterial infections. The occurrence of immunity and its effectiveness varies greatly in different host animals and against different parasites.[4]

Natural and acquired immunity is now generally considered to play an important part in reducing the damage done by parasites.

[4] Readers interested in a more extensive or more technical discussion of immunity to parasites than that given here are referred to the extensive literature reviewed in citations *6, 14, 19, 21.*

Since it does not afford complete protection, however, and adequate methods of artificial immunization are lacking, it would seem safest and wisest for the livestock producer not to depend on it for prevention of parasitic losses. Instead it would seem highly advisable for him to attempt to prevent and remove parasitic infection wherever possible through sanitation and treatment and to foster the good health of his animals in all possible ways. He would thus not only greatly lessen the necessity for protective reactions but would insure their having the highest effectiveness when mobilized to combat the comparatively small amount of parasitic infection which he may be unable otherwise to control.

The great importance of protective mechanisms in the control of parasitic disease can perhaps be best illustrated by outlining what usually happens under natural conditions when susceptible animals are placed in contact with parasitized ones. The new arrivals will, in general, be protected against the parasites of other unrelated kinds of animals by what is known as natural immunity. For example, hogs will not become infected, even though exposed to infection, with the parasites of horses, and vice versa. Older stock not previously exposed to infection may also be protected by what is known as age immunity. This form of natural immunity is of widespread occurrence. It is especially marked in dogs and cats against hookworms and in chickens against gapeworms. Some of the animals will also be innately more immune than others because of the possession of an inherited individual, species, or breed immunity. For example, Rhode Island Red and Plymouth Rock chickens have been found to be more resistant to certain experimental infections than Leghorns, Buff Orpingtons, and Minorcas (*1*) and in mixed flocks of sheep Cheviots were found more tolerant of parasitism than Leicesters (*6*).

Susceptible animals introduced into an infected environment may be expected to acquire infection and suffer from parasitic injury. As a result their natural mechanisms of defense are stimulated to repair the damage and to counteract the presence of the parasites. Multiplication of the parasites in the blood or tissues or their increase through continual exposure to new infection forces the animals to react more vigourously to the increasing number of parasites. If the number of parasites increases more rapidly than the activity of the protective reactions, the animals suffer and perhaps die from the effects of severe parasitism. If the number of parasites is small or increases slowly, the defense forces of the animals have time to become mobilized and may produce an acquired immunity.

This type of immunity has been shown to develop in many different kinds of animals and with many parasitic infections under both experimental and natural conditions. Especially interesting studies have been made of acquired immunity in cattle against cattle tick fever (*16*); in birds, against malaria (*20*); in sheep, against stomach worms (*18*); and in laboratory animals, against ticks.

The maintenance of a high level of general health is regarded as important in promoting immunity to parasitism. Such factors as the presence of bacterial disease, multiple parasitic infection, hemorrhage, and the extra demands of breeding, gestation, and lactation have all been cited as detrimental. Inadequate and deficient diets have also been shown to lessen immunity. For example, it has been shown that both natural and acquired immunity to hookworm infection breaks down when immune dogs are fed a generally deficient diet (*8*); that chickens on diets deficient in vitamins A, B, and D become more susceptible to infection with the common intestinal roundworm (*2, 3, 4*); and that whereas a diet deficient in vitamin A increases susceptibility to infestation with lice, a diet containing an abundance of this vitamin will prevent or cure such infestation (*15*).

When the parasites and the injuries they cause are localized in one particular part of the body, blood cells and circulating antibodies are mobilized at that point by the process of inflammation. Although this process occurs in all animals during the course of the primary infection, it is much more rapid and more marked in an immune animal. The harmful products of the parasites are precipitated, neutralized, and destroyed by the cells and fluid of the inflammatory exudate (material discharged), such as pus. The larger, many-celled parasites may also ingest the exudate and be subjected to its action internally as well as externally. Evidence of such action may be seen in the formation of precipitates in the intestine and on the outside of parasites immobilized in the tissues of immune animals.

After the parasites have become inactive and their development has been checked, they are gradually hemmed in by densely packed cells, which form nodules or cysts that become fibrous by the gradual formation of scar tissue around them. The parasite is imprisoned until it dies and is either gradually dissolved by the surrounding macrophages or persists as a calcified, or hardened, remnant. Meanwhile, the tissues injured by the parasite are being repaired by the replacement of destroyed cells and by scar-tissue formation.

The general mechanism of immunity outlined in this brief description is probably of wide occurrence since it has been observed with such diverse parasites as fly maggots, tapeworm larvae, and the larvae of roundworms. The basic phenomenon involved-interference with the normal feeding and development of the parasite by a protective substance in the animal–is probably also operative in immunity against parasites which are essentially outside the tissues. This has been demonstrated in the case of ticks and intestinal worms. Antibodies are evidently of primary importance in these cases of acquired immunity to metazoan parasites, since it has been shown that the immunity can be transferred to a normal animal by the injection of immune serum.

Nutrition and Disease Resistance

Generally speaking, poor nutrition tends to break down the natural barriers of the animal organism against the ravages of the infecting agents of disease. The whole question of how this is accomplished is an exceedingly complex one. Infections vary widely in their nature, they involve various parts of the body, the many structures are affected differently, and their proper nutrition or repair calls for different food elements. Determining the specific functions of the food constituents has challenged the skill of many investigators. In recent years the vitamins have received major attention, but the various essential mineral elements, the proteins, and the energy intake have also been the subject of research, especially with a view to correcting deficiencies.

Much of the experimental work on the relation of nutrition to resistance has been done on laboratory animals such as the rat, guinea pig, and pigeon. Relatively little attention has been given to farm animals. Because of species differences in the need for several vitamin factors, generalizations from the results with laboratory animals are not necessarily applicable to cattle, sheep, swine, and horses.

The need of the higher animals for vitamin A and the early work which showed a close association of bacterial infection with xerophthalmia, a serious nutritional disease due to lack of vitamin

A, have naturally focused attention on this factor. Vitamin A has been properly termed the "anti-infective factor." It has been suggested that the underlying cause for the increased susceptibility of vitamin-A-deficient animals resides in the changes produced in the epithelial tissues (those of the skin and lining membranes) through the substitution of keratinized, or horny, tissue for normal tissue. This change occurs in the respiratory, alimentary, and genitourinary tracts, the eye, and the glands of the throat and ear. If this is the case, the change in epithelial tissues brought about by lack of vitamin A increases the susceptibility to invasion by disease-producing organisms, but there is not necessarily a decrease of immunity in the strictly medical sense. Certain experiments in which the disease organisms were artificially injected into the animal have demonstrated that the decrease in resistance is due to more than the mere break-down of epithelial tissue. Animals that received an adequate supply of vitamin A in their food were much less susceptible to the disease produced by the injection of the infecting agent than were the deficient animals.

All farm animals require vitamin A, and a number of reports are available on experimental work on the association of the deficiency and disease resistance. There is considerable evidence that the incidence of white scours in calves is associated with vitamin A; thus Stewart and McCallum (*17*) found that a lowered vitamin A content in the colostrum of the cow was associated with an increased number of deaths among calves infected with *Bacillus coli*. It does not necessarily follow that all cases of white scours will respond to vitamin A therapy. Some persons have suspected that increased resistance to tuberculosis was associated with adequate vitamin A intake, but a limited amount of work with pigs has not brought out such a relationship. Cattle maintained on a vitamin-A-deficient diet have appeared to be more susceptible to infections and have shown a relatively high mortality rate as compared with animals fed on adequate rations.

The evidence on the influence of vitamin D on infection is conflicting. Experimental findings with laboratory animals fed on diets that produced rickets have indicated a decreased resistance to certain micro-organisms and no change in resistance to other organisms.

It has been established that the needs of herbivoures for the factors of the vitamin B complex are or can be met for the most part through synthesis of the vitamin factors by micro-organisms residing in the alimentary tract. Swine and poultry, however, depend upon the diet for these factors. Experimental work on vitamin B_1 deficiency has shown that animals so affected are generally less resistant to infection and succumb more readily to the ravages of disease than normal animals. It is believed that the lowered body temperature and possibly the loss of appetite resulting from a prolonged intake of the vitamin-B_1-deficient diet is largely responsible. The pronounced fall in body temperature that may occur is well illustrated in studies on pigs (22), in which a drop of as much as 8° F. was recorded. From the standpoint of loss of appetite, a decrease in the power of the blood to promote the formation of phagocytes (devouring cells), which occurs in starvation, as established by the work of Gellhorn and Dunn (*9*), may well account for the decreased resistance.

Evidence is accumulating that necrotic enteritis in swine, a disease produced by *Salmonella suipestifer* and possibly other related organisms, can be alleviated by the use of nicotinic acid. The fact that liver and certain other natural feedstuffs are more effective than nicotinic acid in effecting cures or in preventing the disease suggests that other factors besides nicotinic acid are involved. The mode of action is not understood, but there appears to be an increase in the building of scar tissue over the lesions of dead tissue in the intestine.

The quality and quantity of protein in the diet are thought to bear a close relation to the resistance of human beings to certain infective diseases. The unusual food habits of certain primitive tribes or of groups of people on restricted diets in wartime have been cited to show that a decreased protein intake was associated with an increase in the occurrence and severity of infectious diseases such as tuberculosis. Lowered protein intake apparently reduced the resistance to certain infections in dogs and in suckling pigs. On the other hand McCay and others (*11*) have reported that moderate restriction in the food intake of rats, sufficient to retard their growth and development but prolonging their span of life, lessened their susceptibility to lung disease at approximately 1 year of age, when normal rats suffered severely. Well-founded evidence is available to show that lowered incidence of middle-ear and lung disorders is found among retarded animals.

A lowered intake of protein and calcium by sheep kept on poor pasture has been suspected of contributing to a decrease, below the normal levels, in the amounts of the normal lysins (substances capable of dissolving bacteria) of *Bacillus coli* and *B. suipestifer*, and of the agglutinins (substances capable of causing the clumping of bacteria) of *Brucella abortus* and *B. paratyphosus*.

On the other hand, studies on the relation of diet to infectious abortion by Hart, Hadley, and Humphrey (*10*) showed that a good ration well fortified with protein, fat, calcium, phosphorus, and iodine did not increase resistance to inoculation with *Brucella abortus* over that shown by heifers fed a so-called poor ration. The authors observed that vitamin A was an important cause of failure in reproduction. Where the restriction is so severe that it approaches starvation conditions there seems to be little doubt that the resistance of the body to infection is decreased. The Colorado Agricultural Experiment Station (*13*) has found that sheep deprived of feed for short periods are subject to paratyphoid dysentery. It appeals that the organism *Salmonella aertrycke* is a normal resident of the intestinal tract and develops added virulence under certain conditions, among which deprivation of feed is one.

The general belief is that both the normal antibodies of the serum and the power to form antibodies are not affected by dietary deficiencies. Even this premise may be contradicted, however, as evidence accumulates on the corrective and stimulative action of food factors in the formation of antibodies.

The examples presented in the relationship of nutrition and disease resistance in farm animals are intended to show, on the one hand, the nature of the relationship and, on the other, the scarcity of conclusive data. In spite of the latter, there can be little doubt that nutritive well-being in general is essential for the animal body to combat and counteract the action of disease-producing organisms. The fact that a certain nutritive essential does not appear to bear a direct relation to resistance to a particular infectious disease should not be taken as proof of a lack of relationship.

Literature Cited

(1) ACKERT, J.E., EISENBRANDT, L.L., WILMOTH, J.H., and others (1935). COMPARATIVE RESISTANCE OF FIVE BREEDS OF CHICKENS TO THE NEMATODE ASCARIDIA LINEATA (SCHNEIDER). Jour. Agr. Res. 50: 607- 624, illus.

(2) _______McILVAINE, MARIAN FISHER, and CRAWFORD, NAOMI ZIMMERMAN (1931). RESISTANCE OF CHICKENS TO PARASITISM AFFECTED BY VITAMIN A. Amer. Jour. Hyg. 13: 320-336.

(3) _______and NOLF, L.O. (1931). RESISTANCE OF CHICKENS TO PARASITISM AFFECTED BY VITAMIN B. Amer. Jour. Hyg. 13: 337-344, illus.

(4) _______and SPINDLER, LLOYD A. (1929). VITAMIN D AND RESISTANCE OF CHICKENS TO PARASITISM. Amer. Jour. Hyg. 9: 292-307.

(5) BUNYEA, HUBERT (1939). USE OF THE RAPID WHOLE-BLOOD TEST FOR PULLORUM DISEASE. U.S., Dept. Agr. Misc. Pub. 349, 18 pp., illus.

(6) CAMERON, THOMAS, W.M. (1935). IMMUNITY AGAINST ANIMAL PARASITES. 12th Internatl. Vet. Cong. (1934) Proc. 3: 44-65.

(7) EICHHORN, A., and CRAWFORD, A.B. (1941). BRUCELLOSIS OF CATTLE (BANG'S DISEASE, INFECTIOUS ABORTION). U.S. Dept. Agr. Farmers' Bul. 1871, 21 pp., illus.

(8) FOSTER, A.O., and CORT, W.W. (1935). FURTHER STUDIES ON THE EFFECT OF A GENERALLY DEFICIENT DIET UPON THE RESISTANCE OF DOGS TO HOOKWORM INFESTATION. Amer. Jour. Hyg. 21: 302-318, illus.

(9) GELLHORN, ERNST, and DUNN, J.O. (1937). UNDERNUTRITION, STARVATION AND PHAGOCYTOSIS. Jour. Nutr. 14: 145-153, illus.

(10) HART, E.B., HADLEY, F.B., and HUMPHERY, G.C. (1932). THE RELATION OF NUTRITION TO CONTAGIOUS CATTLE ABORTION. Wis. Expt. Sta. Res. Bul. 112, 45 pp., illus.

(11) McCAY, C.W., ELLIS, G.H., BARNES, LEROY L., and others (1939). CHEMICAL AND PATHOLOGICAL CHANGES IN AGING AND AFTER RETARDED GROWTH. Jour. Nutr. 18: 15-25, illus.

(12) MOHLER, JOHN R., and EICHHORN, ADOLPH (1911). THE DIAGNOSIS OF GLANDERS BY COMPLEMENT FIXATION. U.S. Bur. Anim. Indus. Bul. 136, 31 pp., illus.

(13) NEWSOM, I.E., and THORP, FRANK, JR. (1938). LAMB DISEASES IN COLORADO FEEDLOTS. Colo. Expt. Sta. Bul. 448, 42 pp., illus.

(14) SANDGROUND, J.H. (1929). A CONSIDERATION OF THE REPLATION OF HOST-SPECIFICITY OF HELMINTHS AND OTHER METAZOAN PARASITES TO THE PHENOMENA OF AGE RESISTANCE AND ACQUIRED IMMUNITY. Parasitology 21: [227]-255.

(15) SEARLS, ED. M., and SNYDER, FRED M. (1939). A STUDY OF THE RELATION OF VITAMIN A TO LOUSE RESISTANCE IN RATS. Jour. Parasitol. 25: 425-430.

(16) SMITH, THEOBALD, and KILBOURNE, F.L. (1893). INVESTIGATIONS INTO THE NATURE, CAUSATION AND PREVENTION OF TEXAS OR SOUTHERN CATTLE FEVER. U.S. Bur. Anim. Indus. Bul. 1, 301 pp., illus.

(17) STEWART, JAMES, and McCALLUM, JENNIE WHITELAW (1938). "WHITE SCOUR" IN CALVES AND RELATED INFECTIONS. I. THE SIGNIFICANCE OF THE VITAMIN A CONTENT OF THE COLOSTRUM As A PREDISPOSING FACTOR IN THE CAUSATION OF SUCH CONDITIONS. Jour., Compar. Path. and Ther. 51: 290-295.

(18) STOLL, NORMAN R. (1929). STUDIES WITH THE STRONGYLOID NEMATODE, HAEMONCHUS CONTORTUS. I. ACQUIRED RESISTANCE OF HOSTS UNDER NATURAL REINFECTION CONDITIONS OUT-OF-DOORS, Amer. Jour. Hyg. 10: 384-418, illus.

(19) TALIAFERRO, WILLIAM H. (1929). THE IMMUNOLOGY OF PARASITIC INFECTIONS. 414 pp., illus. New York and London.

(20) _______ (1931). THE MECHANISM OF ACQUIRED IMMUNITY IN AVIAN MALARIA. South. Med. Jour. 24: 409-415, illus.

(21) _______ (1940). THE MECHANISM OF ACQUIRED IMMUNITY IN INFECTIONS WITH PARASITIC WORMS. Physiol. Revs. 20: 469-492.

(22) VAN ETTEN, CECIL, ELLIS, N.R., and MADSEN, L.L. (1940). STUDIES ON THE THIAMIN REQUIREMENT OF YOUNG SWINE. Jour. Nutr. 20: 607-625, illus.

Chapter 4

THE ENDOCRINE GLANDS IN HEALTH AND DISEASE

A.H. Frank[1]

[1] *A.H. Frank is Associate Veterinarian, Animal Disease Station, Beltsville, Md., Bureau of Animal Industry.*

Some of the most extraordinary discoveries of modern medicine are those concerned with the endocrine glands and the hormones they secrete. These glands act as a complicated, delicate set of controls over many vital bodily processes. Some of the hormones have remarkable results, both experimentally and in medical practice, and the future win undoubtedly see further developments.

In a normal body the endocrine glands with their secretions function as a very delicately balanced mechanism. An excessive or deficient secretion of one or more of these glands may lead to an abnormal or diseased condition. Many such conditions are now recognized, several of which, such as diabetes, goiter, cretinism, and sexual impotency, may be successfully treated. This is true of man more than of animals. Some secretions are also being studied with the expectation of increasing certain desirable bodily functions beyond what is considered normal.

All animals have endocrine glands. There are nine of them: The pituitary gland, which is located at the base of the brain; the pineal body, also in the brain; the thyroid, parathyroid, and thymus glands, located in the neck; the adrenal glands, in the abdominal cavity near each kidney; the pancreas, also in the abdominal cavity; and the testicles in the male and ovaries in the female. Because the secretions of these glands are emptied directly into blood vessels within themselves, instead of passing through excretory ducts as in ordinary glands, they are also known as ductless glands or glands of internal secretion.

Each of the endocrine glands secretes one or more substances called endocrines, or hormones. The secretions are usually in very minute quantities and are normally formed as needed through nervous impulse or the direct action of one endocrine upon a gland secreting another endocrine. In particular, the hormones control sexual growth and the various stages of reproduction.[2]

The functions of some of the endocrine glands have been recognized for years, but only recently have the particular stimulating substances been recovered from them in pure chemical form. The Bible refers to castrated men (eunuchs), and the changes in physical make-up and behaviour following castration are commonly known; in animal husbandry it is common practice to castrate young bulls, rams, boars, and roosters to improve the tenderness and tastiness of the meat. But the extraction from the testicles of the hormone responsible for male physical characteristics was first made in chemical form in 1935.[3] The action of this substance is proved by the fact that continued treatment of castrated animals and men with it results in the return of male characteristics and conformation.

As will be noted in the following description of the various endocrine glands and their functions, the actions and interactions of the various hormones are very complex. Though much has been learned about the nature of the endocrines during the last 15 years, only a beginning has been made in the discovery and application of remedies involving them. This is due in part to the difficulty of obtaining many of these substances in pure form in sufficient

---

[2] ALLEN, EGDAR. ed. SEX AND INTERNAL SECRETIONS: A SURVEY OF RECENT RESEARCH, 1346 pp., illus. Baltimore. 1939.

[3] BUTENANDT, ADOLF, and HANISCH, GUNTER, UBER TESTOSTERON. UMWANDLUNG DES DEHYDRO-ANDROSTERONS IN ANDROSTENDIOL AND TESTOSTERON; EIN WEG ZUR DARSTELLUNG DES TESTOSTERONS AUS CHOLESTERIN. Hoppe-Seylers Ztschr. f. Physiol. Chem. 237: 89-97, illus. 1935.

quantities for extended experimentation, since the endocrines are not stored in the glands but are formed as needed and released immediately. Since the various hormones are fortunately identical in all animal species, these substances can be obtained from animals killed in abattoirs.

In view of its past accomplishments and the vast amount of work being done at present, endocrinology holds promise of great achievements in the future, especially in the purification and possible synthetic preparation of hormones and their application in medical treatment.

The Pituitary Gland

The pituitary gland is unquestionably the master gland of the body. It consists of two parts, a larger anterior lobe and a smaller posterior lobe. It is located at the base of the brain in a bony cavity and is surrounded by a rich supply of blood vessels.

In the cow it is about 1 inch in diameter and in the rat about 1/16 of an inch. Its secretions are protein in nature and are so complex that chemists have not been able to analyze them. The anterior lobe is the master part. Eleven or more secretions have been attributed to it alone.

Secretions from the Anterior Lobe

Gonadotropic Hormones

The development of such sex characteristics as body conformation and voice, and in the female the estrus cycle, which includes the ripening of the ovum, or egg, in the ovary and its passage into the uterus, or womb, is directly or indirectly the result of stimulation by hormones secreted by the anterior lobe of the pituitary gland. Two of these are the gonadotropic hormones, so-called because they act on the gonads (ovaries the female and testicles in the male). They are known as the follicle-stimulating principle, or prolan A, and the luteinizing principle, or prolan B.

The ovary contains thousands of minute eggs, and during the first half of each estrus cycle one or more of these is developed through the action of the follicle-stimulating hormone. A covering is formed around the egg, and the whole is called a follicle. As the follicle grows in size its expansion is in the direction of the periphery, or outside of the ovary. Its growth is characterized by an increase in the quantity of fluid, and when mature it has the appearance of a large blister protruding from the surface of the ovary. After ripening, one of two things may happen to the follicle:

(1) Normally, the follicle is ruptured by the action of the other gonadotropic hormone, the luteinizing principle, and the ovum is set free to advance into the uterus. After the escape of the ovum from the follicle, the latter becomes filled with yellowish cells and is thereafter known as the corpus luteum, or yellow body. The luteinizing hormone derives its name from the corpus luteum, which it stimulates directly.

(2) Abnormally, the follicle may fail to rupture, developing into a cyst. The cyst may remain stationary or increase in size. Other follicles generally develop similarly, and their walls become thickened. The follicular fluid (containing estrogenic hormone, described later) in these cysts may change the normal reproductive cycle to frequent or constant heat. Cystic ovaries, if treated early, may be benefited by the gonadotropic hormones; but chronic cases do not respond satisfactorily to such treatment, and the cysts may have to be broken down mechanically. Sometimes the cysts reform and must again be ruptured. Ovariectomy, or removal of the ovary, is recommended in persistent cases.

An excess of luteinizing hormone may act on an immature follicle to stimulate the production of a corpus luteum before rupture occurs, thus preventing the subsequent release of the egg.

In males the luteinizing principle stimulates the cells in the testicle to secrete the male sex hormone. The luteinizing hormone is predominant in the urine of pregnant women from about the eighth day after missing the last menstrual period to parturition. A test for its presence makes possible the early detection of pregnancy.

After ovulation in the female, if fertilization occurs, the corpus luteum remains active until pregnancy is ended, but if not, it gradually disappears. No further heat periods occur until the corpus luteum has become inactive. In cattle its disappearance is sometimes sluggish and it must be expelled by pressure of the hand on the ovary before the cow can again come in heat. The luteinizing hormone activates the corpus luteum, and the latter in turn secretes hormones that act directly on the uterus and indirectly on the mammary glands, described later.

In addition to initiating ovogenesis (ripening of the germ cells in the ovaries of females) and maintaining this ovarian germ-cell activity, the follicle-stimulating principle, prolan A, initiates spermatogenesis (ripening of the germ cells, or spermatozoa, of the testicles) in young males and maintains this activity in mature males. It is used in man and animals to overcome some types of sterility.

When extracts containing this follicle-stimulating hormone are injected into sexually immature animals, precocious sexual maturity is produced. Ovaries of infantile female rats may be increased in weight 10 to 20 times in 96 hours. Young children who suffer from a tumor involving the pituitary, which causes an excessive secretion of this hormone, may reach sexual maturity at 5 years of age or younger.

Between the 42nd, and 120th days of pregnancy, the blood of pregnant mares is rich in this principle, and a physiological test of their blood serum for the presence of this hormone may be used to determine whether pregnancy exists.

Various prepatations rich in gonadotropic principles have been used to overcome sexual sluggishness, especially in active gonads, in mature animals. Ewes may be brought into estrus with serum from pregnant mares or with pituitary extracts and bred during their non-breeding season. Some types of sterility in women and animals can be successfully treated with this extract. Over dosage may result in the ripening of abnormally large numbers of eggs. This is undesirable, as there is not enough space in the female reproductive tract for a large number of fetuses to develop, and abortion or mummification of a number of them may follow.

Mammogenic Hormone

The gonadotropic hormones indirectly stimulate the pituitary to secrete other hormones. As already noted, their action upon the ovary stimulates the growth of the follicle and the corpus luteum, and these in turn secrete the two female sex hormones. One action of the female sex hormones is the direct stimulation of the pituitary to secrete the mammogenic principle. The mammogenic principle directly stimulates the growth and development of the mammary gland, in which milk is secreted and stored. The hormone is secreted during each estrus cycle and produces some growth of the mammary gland; but following conception it is secreted continuously and stimulates the complete development of the mammary gland for that gestation period. If an unlimited supply of this hormone were available, it might be possible to grow large udders on all cows.

Lactogenic Hormone

At parturition, or delivery of young, there is a rapid reduction in the secretion of the sex hormones. This may furnish the stimulus which activates the pituitary to secrete the lactogenic, or milk-stimulating, principle.

The lactogenic hormone initiates milk secretion in the completely developed mammary gland. Both males and females of most species of mammals may be brought to full lactation by injections of this hormone when their mammary glands have been experimentally developed. The stimulus for continued milk secretion is maintained by this hormone. Injections into cows in declining lactation resulted in a pronounced increase in milk and butterfat,[4] but this added stimulus is only of short duration.

Growth Hormone

Experimental evidence and observations of certain disease conditions indicate that the pituitary directly influences the growth of animals. By injecting pituitary extracts that contain the active growth principle into growing mice, it is possible to double the normal mature size of the animals.

Pathological conditions of the pituitary, such as tumorous growths, may result in an excessive secretion of the growth hormone. When this occurs in immature animals they grow abnormally large. If it occurs before maturity in man, gigantism (abnormal tallness, 8 feet or over) may be the result. In adults, it produces the condition known as acromegaly, a chronic disease characterized by enlargement of the bones and soft parts of the hands, feet, and face. Retardation of pituitary activity or the destruction of the gland by X-ray checks these conditions, and the injection of sufficient pituitary extract will maintain normal life.

---

[4] FOLLEY, S.J., and YOUNG, F.G. THE EFFECT OF CONTINUED TREATMENT WITH ANTERIOR PITUITARY EXTRACTS ON MILK VOLUME AND MILK-FAT PRODUCTION IN THE LACTATING COW. Biochem. Jour. 33: 193-197, illus. 1939.

It is fairly evident that the secretion of the growth hormone in normal individuals is controlled through heredity. Inherited characters are transmitted through genes in the female egg and the male sperm cell. The gene responsible for growth of the cells of the pituitary that secrete this hormone may be absent, as has been shown in a colony of dwarf mice. The dwarfism was shown to be due to a single recessive character, dependent upon a single gene. Through microscopic study of the pituitary tissues of these mice in comparison with those of normal mice, it was found that certain cells of the pituitary were absent in the dwarfs. When pituitaries from normal mice were transplanted into these dwarfs they made normal growth. Growth also occurred when the growth hormone extract was injected into the dwarfs.[5] This condition can occur in both man and animals cases of human pituitary infantilism or dwarfism occur frequently where the pituitary has been destroyed by disease processes. The injection of pituitary extracts containing the growth principle in proper amounts restores normal growth in these individuals.

The importance of careful selection of individual animals for breeding purposes is clearly seen, since the quantity of growth hormone secreted by an immature animal evidently determines the rate and extent of its growth. In the future it may be possible to run a quantitative test for the growth hormone and eliminate undesirable animals at birth.

Other Anterior-Lobe Hormones

There is evidence that the anterior lobe of the pituitary gland may secrete an active principle (parathyrotropic hormone) that influences the activity of the parathyroids in calcium metabolism.

The outer, or cortical, portion of the adrenal glands (to be described later), which is essential to the maintenance of life, is under the influence of the adrenotropic hormone of the pituitary gland. In animals with the pituitary removed, the cortical portion of the adrenal glands becomes inactive.

Carbohydrate metabolism is known to be influenced by a hormone secreted by the pituitary. Following injections of active pituitary extracts the blood sugar increases considerably, while

---

[5] SMITH, PHILIP E., and McDOWELL, E.C. AN HEREDITARY ANTERIOR-PITUITARY DEFICIENCY IN THE MOUSE. Anat. Rec. 46: 249-257, illus., 1930.

removal of the pituitary causes the blood sugar to fall 50 percent below normal. Some forms of obesity (those in which people weigh 600 pounds or more) are attributed to glandular dysfunctions or upsets, especially dysfunctions of the anterior pituitary.

There are indications that the digestion and assimilation of fats and proteins may be influenced by anterior-pituitary hormones.

An anterior-pituitary principle (the thyrotropic hormone) activates the thyroid gland to secrete the thyroid hormone, thyroxine, described later. In men and animals with the pituitary removed the thyroid becomes inactive.

The secretion of insulin by the pancreas is influenced by the pituitary. In most animals and in man, the disease diabetes mellitus, with its characteristic symptoms of an increased excretion of urine of high sugar content, can be artificially produced by removal of the pancreas. If the pituitary is also removed, the sugar level approaches normal; but if pituitary extract is injected into an animal without the pancreas or pituitary the original condition of excess sugar is again produced. The addition of pituitary extract to insulin has improved the general well-being of some diabetic people.

Secretions from the Posterior Lobe

Pituitrin Hormone

The posterior lobe of the pituitary secretes the hormone pituitrin. Pituitrin may be split into two active principles, both of which act to contract the smooth muscles of the body. One, oxytocin, stimulates the uterus to contraction. Its action is variable, and it is effective in some mammals only near the end of pregnancy. It is used in difficult labour cases to initiate or to increase the power of uterine contractions. If too much is given, the contractions may be too severe and persistent.

The other principle, vasopressin, activates the muscular tissue of the capillaries and arterioles, or small blood vessels, and thus induces a rise in blood pressure. It increases peristalsis, the wavelike motion of the intestines, by contracting the intestinal muscles. In the dairy cow, it is responsible for the letting down of the milk. Manipulation of the udder and teats at the beginning of milking stimulates the release of this hormone. By contracting the muscles of the udder, it forces the milk into the larger milk channels and cisterns, where it can be readily removed. Its stimulus is short-lived, so a fast milker can obtain more milk than a slow one.

The kidneys are influenced directly by the posterior lobe through its stimulation of the filtering mechanism. Removal or destruction of the posterior pituitary leads to the disease diabetes insipidus, a chronic condition marked by great thirst and passage of large amounts of urine with no excess of sugar.

The Testicle

The testicle has two major functions:

(1) Production of spermatozoa, which is seasonal in the majority of animals but continuous in man, monkey, and most of the domestic animals; and

(2) The secretion of the male sex hormone, testosterone. In most species, with the exception of birds, the testicles are located in the scrotum, which is outside of the body cavity proper. As previously stated, their activities are under the direct influence of the pituitary.

Testosterone Hormone

The testicles begin to secrete testosterone actively at the time of puberty, or sexual maturity. This hormone induces the development of secondary sex characters and stimulates the accessory male sex glands, the prostate, seminal vesicles, and Cowper's gland. Small or infantile genitalia of immature and mature men may be grown to normal size or larger by the injection of this hormone, and in some cases fertility is restored in sterile males by the simultaneous injection of prolan A.

Sexual desire may be enhanced in subnormal and castrated males by the injection of this hormone. Its continuous injection into castrates enables them to perform the copulatory act successfully and restores the characteristic secondary sex characters in long-standing cases. It also tends to correct the castration atrophy (drying up) of the adrenal glands and restores them to normal condition.

Testosterone has been chemically analyzed and synthesized, so that it is available in pure form. It has been used successfully in correcting cryptorchidism (failure of the testicle to descend into the scrotum) in boys and young men; testicles not descending during such treatment are generally retained by mechanical impediments. It is antagonistic to the female sex hormone, estrogen, which induces heat and female characteristics in the female. The injection of testosterone will prevent heat, and prolonged injections produce male characteristics in normal females.

Ovaries

The ovaries, two in number, are the reproductive glands of the female. They are located in the abdominal cavity, one on each side, and are connected to the uterus, or womb, by a tube which serves as a passage channel for the eggs, or ova. Their functions are threefold:

(1) Production of the egg;

(2) Production of the follicle, which secretes the female sex hormone, estrogen; and

(3) Production of the corpus luteum, which secretes the other female sex hormone, progestin.

In normal females ovarian activity which is under the influence of the anterior pituitary, is exhibited in rhythmic cycles, subject to interruption by pregnancy.

Estrogen Hormone

The fluid within the ovarian follicles of normal females and the blood, urine, and amniotic fluid (contained in the sac that surrounds the embryo) of pregnant mammals are rich sources of estrogen. Small traces have also been detected from other sources. Estrogen has been analyzed chemically and prepared synthetically.

In the non-pregnant female estrogen is secreted by the developing follicle, previously described, during half of the estrus cycle (the changes that take place from the beginning of one heat period to the beginning of the next). Ripening of the follicle and the height of estrogen production is characterized by the onset of heat in the female. It also induces a new growth of the epithelium, or lining cells, of the uterus and vagina. A deficiency of estrogen is manifest in some animals. A large percentage of mares are known to pass through estrus cycles without showing signs of heat, although ovulation (releasing of the egg) occurs at the normal time, as proved by mares becoming pregnant following artificial insemination.

Estrogen induces the development of the secondary sex characters of the female, about the most noticeable of which are the characteristic plumage of birds and a certain refinement of stature and features in some mammals. During the cycle, as already indicated, it stimulates the pituitary to secrete mammogen to a limited extent.

In most animals the egg or eggs are expelled from the ovary during or immediately following estrus. Primates (man and monkey) do not outwardly express estrus, but their reproductive tracts pass through similar cyclic changes. Estrus may be induced by the injection of estrogen in both normal females that do not come into heat and those with their ovaries removed. It acts directly upon the vagina and uterus, inducing a new epithelial growth similar to that of the normal cycle.

Because of its action on the epithelium, estrogen is used to treat gonorrhea in young girls, and it should be beneficial in diseases that affect the epithelium of the vagina and the uterus of animals. Large injections immediately following conception (fertilization of the egg) will terminate pregnancy. The presence of this hormone during pregnancy inhibits the pituitary from secreting the follicle-stimulating principle.

Progestin Hormone

Immediately following rupture of the follicle, the corpus luteum begins to grow into the follicular cavity under the stimulus of the luteinizing hormone (prolan B) of the pituitary. It immediately begins to secrete progestin, which stimulates an increase in blood supply and further development of the epithelium of the uterus in preparation for implantation or embedding of the egg, if fertilized. Small amounts of estrogen are also secreted, which act with the progestin to further stimulate the pituitary to secrete mammogen. When the male sperm cell unites with the ovum, the latter becomes attached to the wall of the uterus. This implantation of the fertilized egg furnishes a stimulus to the pituitary to secrete prolan B and maintain the corpus luteum for the duration of pregnancy. With advancement of pregnancy, an increase of estrogen, together with the progestin, stimulates the maximum secretion of mammogen, and the mammary gland is completely developed.

In sterile cycles the corpus luteum is short-lived, and the stimulus from estrogen and progestin soon ceases. This is followed by menstruation in primates, while there is no outward sign in other mammals. A new cycle begins with the growth of a new follicle.

Abortions and resorptions (absorption of the embryo) that occur during early pregnancy may be due to a deficiency of progestin. The corpus luteum may be slow to develop and thus fail to prepare the uterus for implantation.

The Parathyroid Glands

The parathyroids are ductless glands that in large animals are about as large as a grain of wheat. They are two to four in number and are located one or two under each lobe of the thyroid gland.

Parathormone is produced by the parathyroids and maintains the equilibrium between the insoluble calcium and phosphorus compounds in the skeleton and the soluble compounds of these essential minerals in the blood. Extracts are used in treating cases of reduced secretion of the hormone (hypoparathyroidism).

The Adrenal Glands

The two adrenal glands are located in the abdominal cavity, one in front of each kidney. They are ductless and consist of two parts, the medullary (inner) and cortical (outer) portions.

The hormone adrenin is secreted by the medullary part of the adrenal glands. Its action is similar to that of pituitrin. It is used extensively in cases of shock as an indirect heart stimulant and to check hemorrhages by contracting the muscles of the small blood vessels.

The hormone cortin, which is essential to the maintenance of life, is contained in the cortical portion of the gland. Extracts of this portion have been used to maintain life in animals after the glands are removed. This hormone is similar to testosterone in its chemical make-up and its antagonistic reaction to estrogen. When tumorous growths of the adrenal glands in young girls cause an excessive secretion, this antagonism to estrogen is demonstrated by the production of male characteristics, such as growth of beard on the face, coarseness of voice, cessation of menstruation, and decreased modesty. The condition is alleviated when the tumor is removed.

Addison's disease, which is characterized by bronzelike pigmentation of the skin, severe prostration, progressive anemia, low blood pressure, diarrhea, and digestive disturbances, is due to a decreased secretion or functioning of the cortical portion of the adrenal gland. The disease can be corrected in most cases by injections of cortin.

The Thyroid

The thyroid is a ductless gland resembling a tiny shield in shape. It is located in front and on both sides of the windpipe. The familiar enlargement in the neck called goiter is an enlargement of this gland.

The thyroid, as stated previously, is stimulated by the pituitary to secrete the hormone thyroxin, which controls the energy output, or metabolism, of the body. Chemical analysis shows that thyroxin contains large amounts of iodine. An increased production of thyroxin gives the individual an excessive amount of energy. The metabolic rate may be doubled by injection of thyroxin. Its injection into rams has been found to activate their sexual functioning and enhance the production of fertile semen during the non-breeding season, summer. Practical use of the method would materially increase the possibility of getting early lamb crops by rendering the rams fertile at an earlier date than their normal breeding season. In hibernating animals the thyroid diminishes in size and practically ceases activity during hibernation. The injection of thyroxin interrupts the hibernal sleep. An overactive gland may be corrected in part by surgical removal of a portion of the tissue.

A decreased secretion of thyroxin makes the individual sluggish. The metabolic rate may be decreased at least half by removal of the gland. Animals born without the thyroid or those in which it becomes inactivated during infancy fail to develop normally in mental, physical, and sexual activity. In children this is known as cretinism. A similar condition in adults is known as myxedema, a disease characterized by the decreased function of the thyroid gland and marked by dropsylike swelling, especially of the face and hands, and a general slowing down or sluggishness. In this condition the gland may become quite small. All cases of cretinism and myxedema are benefited and most cases may be cured by the continuous administration of thyroxin. Feeding the dried gland provides a satisfactory supplement for the normal gland. In some cases of cretinism the addition of the growth principle from the pituitary may prove beneficial.

A deficiency of iodine in the diet may result in a decreased functioning of the thyroid gland. This is discussed in the articles on nutritional diseases in this volume.

The Pancreas

The pancreas is located in a loop of the small intestine adjacent to the stomach. It has a two fold function. It secretes digestive juices, which enter directly into the intestine, and the hormone insulin, which enters the blood stream. Insulin is secreted by small islets of cells scattered throughout the connective tissue of the pancreas.

When the secretion of insulin falls below the normal level or ceases, diabetes mellitus is produced. The carbohydrate metabolism is badly upset, and the patient is unable to utilize sugars, large amounts of which appear in the blood and are eliminated in the urine, which is decidedly increased in volume. Insulin for the treatment of the disease is now available in both crystalline form and water solution.

An over-secretion or an injection of insulin into normal animals results in a decrease of sugar in the blood and if continued will lead to coma. An increase in the blood-sugar concentration appears to be a stimulus for insulin secretion.

The Pineal Gland

The pineal is a ductless gland located in the central part of the brain. Injection of pineal extracts and implants of the gland have no effect on growth and development of normal animals. There is some indication, however, that daily administration of 1 cubic centimeter of pineal extracts to successive generations of rats has resulted in an increase in the frequency of breeding and a retardation in the rate of growth of the offspring.

The Thymus Gland

The thymus is on irregular glandular mass extending from the thyroid gland to the thorax or chest; it is very prominent and well-developed in young animals, especially calves, in which it is called sweetbread. It becomes degenerate at the time of maturity. Experiments performed to establish the action of the thymus on growth and sexual development have led to conflicting results. The majority of workers have found it to be negligible. There is some indication that the offspring of successive generations all of which have received injections of thymus extracts may grow to maturity at a faster rate but do not exceed normal size.

Antihormones

Certain experimental evidence indicates that the hormones may be held in check or inactivated by antihormone principles. For instance, after long-continued injection of prolan B into an animal, the blood serum is found to contain antibodies to this hormone, and the injection of blood from this animal into a normal female will prevent ovulation and the growth of the corpus luteum.

This should be a warning that the wholesale, repeated injection of animals with hormones may aggravate rather than alleviate certain troubles. To apply any hormone treatment successfully, it is first essential to determine the cause of the condition that needs to be corrected and then choose the appropriate treatment. The diagnosis of any hormonal difficulty may be complicated by an unbalanced condition among various hormones as well as by the presence of antibodies.

Chapter 5

THE RELATION OF GENETICS TO DISEASE

Hugh C. McPhee[1]

[1] *Hugh C. McPhee is Chief, Animal Husbandry Division, Bureau of Animal Industry.*

The breeding of disease-resistant varieties of plants is one of the major triumphs of modern genetics. Could disease losses in livestock be reduced in much the same way that production is increased by breeding methods? Here is a cautious yet optimistic viewpoint on a question of great interest to agriculture.

That there is an inherited resistance or susceptibility to diseases is by no means a new concept, but experimental evidence to substantiate the idea is relatively new. In the case of animal diseases, however, practically all the attention has been centered on the disease organisms themselves, the tissue changes brought about by their presence in the host, and therapeutic measures for control. Such studies have been remarkably fruitful in medical science, including veterinary medicine; the extensive use of vaccination as a means of avoiding disease is an example of the importance of the results. Nevertheless, during recent years there has been a growing interest in the natural resistance to disease shown by some individual animals. Interest has been stimulated primarily by advances in genetic knowledge, particularly in relation to physiological characteristics, and by the marked progress made by plant breeders in controlling plant diseases through the development of resistant strains.

The science of genetics seeks to explain the variations in characteristics shown by individuals connected by a common line of ancestry. If disease is defined as any abnormal condition of the body tissues, then inheritance may have a four-way relationship to it. There may be (1) specific inherited resistance to certain infectious diseases, (2) a connection between inherited vigour and resistance, (3) inherent variations in the disease organism itself, giving rise to strains differing in virulence, and (4) various specific abnormalities, many of them lethal. Many such abnormalities have been shown by experimental evidence to be inherited; in fact, there is much more information on this point than on the other three.

Inherited Resistance to Disease

Specific inherited resistance to an infectious disease is perhaps best illustrated by Lambert's[2] experiments with White Leghorn chickens, the object of which was to determine whether continued selection for resistance to fowl typhoid would lower the death loss in the flock. The foundation stock consisted of 220 birds, all of which were given a massive dose of virulent fowl typhoid bacteria. Of this group 47.7 percent died. Among the survivors those showing the least severe clinical symptoms of fowl typhoid were saved as breeders to furnish the first selected generation of chicks. All chicks in this and the four succeeding generations, when 7 days old, were given injections intraperitoneally (into the abdominal lining) of a standard dose of the disease organism. The death losses resulting from these injections for five consecutive generations were 39.8, 29.3, 15.4, 15.0, and 9.4 percent. At the same time the losses in unselected control stock were 89.6, 93.2, 86.2, 86.4, and 85.0 percent. This remarkable difference was brought about by simple selection. It is also of interest that most of the mortality occurred sooner after inoculation in the control lot than in the selected group, indicating all even higher resistance in the latter than the figures for losses show. Following the five generations of selection, matings were made between males selected for resistance and unselected females, and also between selected females and unselected males. The results showed that the

---

2 LAMBERT, W.V. NATURAL RESISTANCE TO DISEASE IN THE CHICKEN. Jour. Immunol. 23: 229-260, illus, 1932.

male as well as the female transmits resistance and that a passive transfer of immunity through the eggs probably is not involved. The death loss among the chicks from the resistant male × unselected female cross was 63.5 percent, while in the reciprocal group (unselected male × resistant female) it was 50.7 percent. These figures are intermediate between those for the selected and the control stocks.

A few other investigators have reported somewhat similar results for other diseases. Schott[3] was able in 6 years of selective breeding to reduce mortality from mouse typhoid from 82 to 24 percent. Roberts[4] developed a strain of chickens which showed only 35 percent mortality from pullorum injection, as compared with 73 percent in an unselected group. A recent case reported from the California Experiment Station concerns the discovery of some pigs that seem to be immune to repeated injections of the *Brucella* organism and to transmit the resistance to their offspring. Only a preliminary report has been made, and more breeding results are needed before it will be known whether or not this is a case of a genetic factor giving practically complete resistance to a specific disease. It is to be hoped that the resistance of these pigs to *Brucella* will prove to be hereditary and that this finding can be used to advantage in combating brucellosis in swine. There have been reports in the past, however, of pigs immune to another disease, hog cholera, but no resistant strain has yet arisen from such animals, and it is entirely possible that such resistance may be due to acquired immunity or to some other factor that confused the genetic picture.

The cases cited show clearly that selective breeding can result in a marked decrease in death losses from certain diseases. If, for example, a loss of 85 to 90 birds out of every 100 can be cut down to 10, it would seem to be a matter of considerable economic importance. Why, then, has a system of selective breeding never been adopted in practice? The answer is probably to be found in the fact that resistance so secured is difficult and expensive to maintain. As Lambert's results show, a single outcross, bringing in other genetic factors, eliminates a large part of the resistance; then the process of selection, including tests with the disease organism, has to be

---

[3] SCHOTT, RALPH. THE INHERITANCE OF RESISTANCE TO SALMONELLA AERTRYCKE IN VARIOUS STRAINS OF MICE. Genetics 17: 203-229, illus, 1932.

[4] ROBERTS, E. INHERITANCE OF RESISTANCE TO DISEASE IN ANIMALS. Internatl. Cong. Genetics Proc. 6(2): 169-170. 1932.

repeated all over again in order to bring the stock back to a reasonably high degree of resistance. All this takes time and money. Unless the livestock industry can use such a system economically, it cannot be expected to find widespread application.

Theoretically, it would seem just as possible, through the application of genetic principles, to cut death losses from disease in half as it is to double egg production by breeding. The fact is, however, that in no single investigation of the possibility of breeding resistance to disease has the work been carried far enough to show how it might be given really practical application.

The plant breeder can hand the farmer seed from resistant plants, and the resulting plants will remain resistant in succeeding generations because their genetic purity is held relatively constant by self-fertilization, which is a natural process for many crop plants, including some of the grains. This the animal breeder cannot do. What can be done with animals is to approximate genetic stabilization through a less intense system of inbreeding than is possible with plants, but one sufficiently intense to fix any heredity for disease resistance that may now exist in a diluted form in animal populations. The problems of distributing resistant stocks to farmers and maintaining resistance afterward are bridges that must be crossed at a later time. The first step is for the experimenter to locate resistance and build up strains that breed reasonably true for this characteristic.

It can be said that such work has been begun only in a very minor way. The method of breeding used by most livestock breeders does not lead quickly to the formation of lines sufficiently inbred to mean much as far as the fixation of heredity for resistance to disease is concerned. Moreover, any selection that is practiced probably would be carried out in the absence of disease, because it is not to the advantage of the breeder to have disease in his herd. Thus any closely bred line developed under such conditions would not show significant resistance to any disease except by pure chance. But it is very easy for the experimenter using modern medical and veterinary methods to infect animals with definite doses of disease organisms or agents and identify individuals possessing resistance. The fact that such procedure may work successfully is well illustrated by the recent report, mentioned earlier, by Cameron, Hughes, and Gregory, of the California station, on genetic resistance of swine to brucellosis. Apparently these workers have located an inbred strain in which some individuals possess resistance to this disease. Resistant × resistant matings have produced pigs showing either a complete immunity or a very high resistance. If this resistance persists through following generations, this inbred line will be the first brucellosis-resistant line of pigs to be developed and may furnish the starting point for controlling the disease by breeding methods.

Vigour versus Resistance

The belief is fairly widespread that a vigourous individual is more resistant to infectious diseases than one less vigorous. It would be logical then to assume that inherited vigour would mean inherited resistance to disease. Whether this is true depends to a large extent on the definition of vigour.

The vigour of a family or line of animals is not inherited as a single unit but as a complex of several units which are largely independent of each other. This was shown by Wright[5] with guinea pigs. Long-continued inbreeding brought about a fixation of genetic factors affecting growth, body size, fertility, the occurrence of certain abnormalities, and resistance to tuberculosis. The differences in the closely inbred lines followed a pattern of independent assortment and fixation of heredity for these characteristics; resistance to tuberculosis, for example, did not show a tendency to be associated with any particular element of vigour. Possessing heredity for the elements of vigour is therefore no guaranty of heredity for disease resistance. Moreover, resistance to one disease does not necessarily have anything to do with resistance to another disease. A possibility coming out of the evidence on the lack of a relationship between resistance and inherited vigour is that heredity for vigour might be combined by suitable breeding methods with that for disease resistance; in other words, there is no reason why breeding cannot be used to raise the general levels of vigour and of resistance to disease at the same time.

Changes in Virulence of Disease Organisms

It is a matter of common knowledge that pathogenic organisms vary considerably in virulence, but not much is known about the

---

[5] WRIGHT, SEWALL, AND LEWIS, P.A. FACTORS IN THE RESISTANCE OF GUINEA PIGS TO TUBERCULOSIS, WITH SPECIAL REGARD TO INBREEDING AND HEREDITY. Amer. Nat. 55: 20-580, illus, 1921.

causes of such variations. They may be due to the effects of a changing environment, or to some inherent change in the organism itself, or to both. The one thing certain is that there are changes.

The fact that such changes occur introduces another complexity into the relation of genetics to disease. If the agent itself can mutate and hybridize, there is almost no end to the possible interactions between the host and the organism. What is interpreted to be an increased resistance might well result from a lower virulence, and vice versa. During the last 10 or 15 years there have been many reports on variability in pathogenic bacteria, but it is still not known whether genetics is playing a decisive role in bringing about such changes. Until new evidence is produced, speculation should be held to a minimum. The very important matter of a varying virulence should not, however, be overlooked; but nothing much can be done about it, nor can the facts be discovered, until the animals on which it is tested are stabilized genetically so that the results can be attributed to variations in the organism rather than in the host. Here is a relatively virgin field that is a challenge to research workers.

Hereditary Defects in Farm Animals

Numerous physical variations that occur among animals should be mentioned here because of their relation to disease. Many of them can be classed as defects, and a high proportion are lethal-that is, they kill the animals inheriting them. In many cases the mode of inheritance of the defects has been worked out by actual breeding experiments.

No attempt will be made here to cite all the references to the scientific literature on the subject. Eaton[6] has published a summary report which includes about 150 literature citations, and the reader is referred to his paper for original sources of information.

Cattle

Achondroplasia

Two types of achondroplasia have been reported, one of which seems to be a dominant and the other a recessive. The dominant form is the cause of the bulldog calves which occur in the Dexter

[6] EATON, O.N. A SUMMARY OF LETHAL CHARACTERS IN ANIMALS AND MAN. Jour. Hered. 28: 320-326. 1937.

breed and some African cattle. The affected calves have very short legs, a large rupture, and a much shortened bulldoglike head. The thyroid gland and kidneys are also markedly affected. Such fetuses are usually aborted during the fourth month of pregnancy. The recessive form, which occurs in Telemark and Holstein cattle, also results in a very short head, deformed jaws, and sometimes a cleft palate. Death occurs a few days after birth.

Acroteriasis Congenita

Characterized by either the absence of all limbs or their development only to elbows and hocks, atrophy of the upper jaw, almost complete absence of the lower jaw, and a cleft palate. The affected calves either are still-born or die shortly after birth. Genetically the defect is a single-factor recessive.

Ankylosis

An ossification, or stiffening, of the joint of the lower jaw, which is shortened. It is reported to occur in Norwegian Lyngdal cattle. What is probably a related form in which there is ossification of all joints and a cleft palate occurs in some German cattle. Both are recessive.

Congenital Dropsy

Probably a single factor which results in an accumulation of water in the subcutaneous tissues (those immediately under the skin) and in the body cavities. Affected individual fetuses are frequently dropped 1 or 2 months prematurely.

Congenital Icthyosis

A recessive factor that causes scaly and cracked skin. This factor may have some relation to the epitheliogenesis imperfecta (imperfect formation of skin) reported in Holstein-Friesian and Jersy cattle. Affected individuals have large hairless patches over the body and defective skin on the legs and the mucous membranes of the mouth and nostrils. The animals are born at term but die from septicemia (a general poisoning of the blood) soon afterward.

Hypotrichosis Congenita

A single-factor recessive which prevents hair development except on muzzle, eyelids, ears, pasterns, and top of tail. Affected calves die very soon after birth. It is reported to occur in Swedish Holsteins.

Impacted Molars

The premolars are impacted in the jaw, and the lower jaw, or mandible, is shortened. Affected calves are born at term but usually die during the first week. The defect is reported to occur among Milking Shorthorn cattle.

Muscle Contracture

A single-factor recessive causing a bending backward of the head, stiff neck, and rigid joints. It is reported to occur among Norwegian and Holstein cattle. A related form in Red Danish cattle makes the hind legs lame so the calf cannot stand. Such calves are born alive but soon die.

Short Spine

A single-factor recessive which occurs in Norwegian mountain cattle. The axial skeleton is much shortened, and the ribs and vertebrae are fused. Affected calves are usually still-born.

Some other lethal defects, such as mummification of fetuses and short limbs, have been reported, but there is some question as to whether they may not be only a phase of the action of one of the other factors already mentioned.

Horses

Atresia Coli

A single-factor recessive which results in death 3 or 4 days after birth. The ascending colon is greatly restricted or has a blind ending. Often the affected individual has a brain tumor.

Abnormal Sex Ratio

A sex-linked recessive factor which kills about one-half of the male colts before birth.

Stiff Forelegs

Characterized by failure to stand and early death, probably due to hereditary factors. Matings between animals known to carry the defect produced 8 crippled to 18 normal foals.

Sheep

Amputated

The absence of hoofs on all four feet. It has been reported to occur in Holland, but the mode of inheritance is unknown.

Earlessness and Cleft Palate

A single-factor recessive which causes cleft palate, earlessness, short lower jaw, and tripartite claws. It has been reported to occur in Norwegian sheep.

Lethal Gray

A recessive factor reported in Turkana sheep in Rumania and in Karakul sheep in Russia. Homozygous gray lambs lie.

Muscle Contracture

A recessive factor which makes leg joints stiff and neck crooked. Lambs are still-born. It is reported to occur in Welsh mountain sheep.

Paralysis

A recessive factor which paralyzes the hind legs and causes death of the affected lamb a few days after birth.

Skeletal Defects

A single-factor recessive, reported to occur among sheep in Iceland, which produces a short body, large skull, short upper jaw, rigid fetlocks, and absence of wool from brisket to anus. The lambs are born alive but soon die.

Swine

Atresia Ani

Partial or complete closure of the anus of pigs. Affected animals die soon after birth. It has been reported in Europe and observed in the United States.

Catlin Mark

A single-factor recessive which causes an opening between the parietal (side) and frontal bones of the head. Death occurs within an hour after birth.

Cleft Palate

A recessive factor which gives various degrees of abnormal palate. Pigs die soon after birth owing to inability to nurse.

Fetal Mortality

A factor, probably recessive, which seems to be associated with inability to utilize certain vitamins and salts, causing death of fetuses.

Hypotrichosis

The hereditary form of hairlessness in swine, which is not lethal as it is in cattle. The most common type of hairlessness in swine is due to an iodine deficiency and usually results in still-born pigs. The administration of iodine to the sow will prevent the occurrence of this type but has no effect on the hereditary form of hairlessness.

Muscle Contracture

A single-factor recessive which causes stiff front legs. Affected individuals are either still-born or die soon after birth.

Paralysis

A single-factor recessive which produces complete paralysis of the hind legs.

Poultry

Abnormal Upper Mandible

A recessive factor which reduces the maxillae (jawbones) and nasal bones and bends the beak to one side. Such chicks rarely hatch.

Chondrodystrophy

Fetal deformation of bones and joints. Inheritance of this defect is complex and probably involves three recessive factors.

Congenital Loco

A single-factor recessive which results in bending back the head and in inability to stand. Over three-fourths of the affected individuals die within a month after hatching.

Creeper

A dominant factor which in homozygous condition causes death on the fourth day of incubation.

Dwarf

A single-factor recessive which causes death when in homozygous combination.

Recessive White

A recessive factor which may be sex-linked. The homozygous whites die.

Short Legs

A factor reported to occur in Dark Cornish fowl which when homozygous causes death near the end of the incubation period.

Sticky Embryo

A recessive factor which causes the presence in the egg of sticky liquids that prevent chicks from hatching.

Crested

An inherited factor which causes extreme cerebral hernia in ducks. Affected individuals die when nearly ready to hatch.

There are some other conditions such as malposition of embryos and embryonic abnormalities of several types, which cause death before hatching, for which the inheritance has not yet been determined.

Conclusions

The preceding list of lethal defects includes those that have been studied sufficiently to determine that they are due to genetic factors. New cases are continually being brought to light as more attention is given to genetic investigations in livestock. For instance, a case of what appears to be inherited hemophilia (delayed clotting of blood), was observed in swine in 1940. This defect is due to a single autosomal recessive factor and thus differs from hemophilia in man, which is sex-linked in its inheritance.

There are some types of defects in small animals, such as guinea pigs and mice, which are known to have a hereditary basis, but which have not been studied in farm animals. An illustration is the well-known case of otocephaly in the guinea pig, which produces cyclopean monsters, with only one eye. The same kind of defect has been observed in cattle, sheep, swine, cats, dogs, and man. While its inheritance is very complex, enough is known to say that herd or flock sires producing it should be discarded.

Fortunately, the number of hereditary lethals occurring among breeds of livestock in the United States is not very great, nor do they appear very often in most stocks. Neveretheless, they are a big factor in some strains, and because most of them are recessive they can be spread far and wide without showing their presence. When lines of ancestry containing such a defect are brought together it may be expected that some of the offspring will show the character. When this occurs it is important to remember that both the sire and the dam carry the recessive genetic factor, and they and all their offspring should be eliminated from the breeding herd if it is desired to get rid of the trouble.

Chapter 6

ARTIFICIAL INSEMINATION AND DISEASE CONTROL

A.H. Frank and Ralph W. Phillips[1]

[1] *A.H. Frank is Associate Veterinarian and Ralph W. Phillips is Senior Animal Husbandman, Bureau of Animal Industry.*

Several livestock diseases are spread either partly or exclusively by contact during breeding. For these, the authors point out, artificial insemination offers an excellent method of control.

The technique of artificial insemination is not new, but only in recent years has it been used on a large scale. Considerable use has been made of it in the Union of Soviet Socialist Republics and other countries. In the United States there is wide interest in the subject; much research is under way, new techniques are being developed, old ones are being improved, and it seems probable that the use of artificial insemination will continue to increase. The most extensive development in the use of artificial insemination in this country has been with dairy cattle; large numbers of cows are now bred to bulls maintained at central points. In March 1941 the number of cows recorded in cooperative artificial-breeding associations for dairy cattle was 70,751, and 237 bulls were being used.[2] The technique

[2] U.S. BUREAU OF DAIRY INDUSTRY. COOPERATIVE DAIRY-CATTLE BREEDING ASSOCIATION. Dairy Herd-Improvement Assoc. Letter 17(3), 29 pp. 1941.

has also been used, less extensively, with beef cattle, horses, sheep, goats, swine, poultry, and fur-bearing animals.

The basic reason for developing artificial insemination has been to increase the usefulness of outstanding sires. There are other advantages of the technique over natural breeding, however, one being that it aids in controlling certain diseases. Many diseases that attack the reproductive organs and glands of animals may be spread by sexual intercourse, and some are transmitted only in this way. Artificial insemination can be used to prevent the spread of a disease from one female to another through the male. If improperly practiced, however, it may be the means of spreading diseases. Most cooperatives obtain the services of a veterinarian for this work, which requires not only a knowledge of the symptoms of diseases but recognition of the necessity for cleanliness, sanitation, and the proper disinfection of utensils before and after use.

Usually in collecting semen from the male, a rubber artificial vagina is used into which the penis is directed when he mounts the female. The semen is collected in a small tube attached to the opposite end of the artificial vagina. There are other methods of collection, but in most cases this is the best for use with mammals. In inseminating the female, a lighted speculum is inserted into the vagina. This illuminates the cervix, into which the semen is injected by means of a long tube attached to a syringe. The technique of collection and insemination in poultry differs from that in mammals because of anatomical differences in the genital tracts. Techniques for both mammals and poultry are described in detail by Lambert and McKenzie.[3]

Semen samples collected from the male in the artificial vagina are subject to contamination with germs or bacteria, just as is milk drawn from the udder. Bacteria in semen may come either from the reproductive organs of the male or from the apparatus used for collection. When the males are healthy, the bacteria are generally harmless to females, but occasionally there may be pus-producing organisms that, if present in excessively large numbers, may temporarily affect the female organs. By such measures as the provision of sanitary surroundings, regular grooming, and the use

---

[3] LAMBERT, W.V. AND McKENZIE, FRED F. ARTIFICIAL INSEMINATION IN LIVESTOCK BREEDING. U.S. Deptt. Agr. Cir. 567, 68 pp., illus., 1940.

of sterile apparatus for collecting, the bacteria in semen from healthy males can be kept down to a very low number, and under such circumstances most types of bacteria do not materially affect fertilizing and keeping qualities.

The male may communicate diseases to the female either mechanically, by carrying the infective organisms from one female to another during mating, or as a result of infection in the reproductive organs. When the disease is communicated mechanically, the infecting organisms are found in the sheath and on the outer surface of the penis. Such cases are especially dangerous, because to all outward appearances the males are healthy and would not be suspected of carrying infection. When the genital organs of the male are actually infected, the organisms are transmitted in the semen, not mechanically. In chronic infections, noticeable swellings may be visible, or the health of the animal may be impaired, and usually his breeding efficiency is greatly reduced or lost. In the early stages of a disease, however, though no impairment of health may be noticeable, the disease-producing organisms may be transferred in the semen to the female.

In most cases of reproductive disorders males contract the disease through sexual contact with infected females; hence the importance of sanitary precautions to prevent the mechanical transfer of infection from one female to another by the instruments, even when the male is absolutely free of disease. It is essential that all instruments be thoroughly cleaned and disinfected after their use on each individual. Chemical disinfectants are generally used for this purpose and may be recommended for all equipment that does not come in direct contact with the semen. As sperm is quickly killed on coming in contact with disinfectants, other means of sterilizing equipment for handling semen must be used. Boiling and sterilization by live steam are the most desirable methods of preparing the applicators and syringes, and sufficient sterile equipment should be provided for each day's work. If only one applicator is available, it should be sterilized before it is used again.

Diseases that may be Controlled through Artificial Insemination

If only males known to be free from disease are selected for semen collection, artificial insemination can play an important part in controlling diseases spread through sexual contact. Among the diseases in this group are granular vaginitis, a disease caused by the organism *Vibrio fetus*, trichomoniasis, navel ill, dourine, brucellosis, coital exanthema, and vent gleet of poultry.

Granular vaginitis is usually a chronic infection of cattle in which the lining of the vagina is attacked by the disease-producing agent. This results in inflammation and the formation of small pustules, which develop a granular appearance. The discharge from an affected cow contains the virus. The external genitals of a bull serving such a cow become contaminated, and he may transmit the disease to other cows in mating.

Vibrio fetus is a micro-organism found at times in the uterus and fetal membranes of pregnant cows and ewes and in the stomach of the fetus. It often causes abortion. It is believed that males may spread the disease during sexual intercourse.

Trichomoniasis is an infection of the genital tract of cows caused by a microparasite. In the female the parasite lodges first in the vagina, where it sets up an irritation and causes a discharge. It may later invade the uterus and cause sterility or abortion during the early stages of pregnancy. It is a true venereal disease transmitted by the male to the female, or vice versa, during mating.

The common condition known as navel ill occurring in foals is produced by a number of different germs. In one type of the disease the sire, in breeding, may transmit the germ to the mare, and the germ then becomes localized in the mare's genital tract. The foal may become infected in the uterus of the dam before birth or outside the uterus at the time of birth.

Dourine, a disease of horses, is similar in many respects to syphilis of man. Stallions become infected from sexual contact with infected mares and spread the disease to other mares. Dourine has been eradicated from most portions of the United States and by the spring of 1942 existed in only a few isolated localities.

Brucellosis of cattle, or Bang's disease, is a disease of the genital organs in both the cow and the bull. It is caused by a germ that is found in vast numbers in the discharge from the uterus of an infected dam following abortion. The bull may become infected in serving an infected cow shortly after she has aborted. In some instances it is possible that the bull, harbouring the germs in his seminal fluid, may transmit the disease directly or indirectly to the cow, but the disease is usually spread in other ways.

In brucellosis of swine, which is similar to the disease in cattle, the germ often becomes localized in the testicles of the boar and is discharged in the seminal fluid. It is possible that sows may become infected in breeding and that boars may become infected when serving infected sows.

Coital exanthema of horses is a venereal disease affecting the external genitalia of mares and stallions. It is transmitted from one sex to the other at breeding time.

In poultry, vent gleet and possibly several other diseases may be spread by the male to the female during sexual intercourse.

Other diseases, such as tuberculosis, may affect the genital organs of male and female animals, but there is no proof of their transmission from one to the other in mating.

The extent to which many diseases are spread through contact during breeding is yet to be determined, but artificial insemination can play a very important part in controlling the diseases which may be spread in this manner. If only healthy sires are used, if sanitary precautions are followed, and if the procedure is entrusted to the care of a qualified and careful practitioner, artificial insemination will break the link in the transmission of genital diseases.

Chapter 7

DISINFECTION AND DISINFECTANTS

F.W. Tilley[1]

[1] *F.W. Tilley is Senior Bacteriologist, Pathological Division, Bureau of Animal Industry.*

When disease breaks out among farm animals, it is often necessary to do a thorough clean-up and disinfecting job to get rid of the infection. Here is practical information about the principal kinds of disinfectants, the advantages and drawbacks of each, and how to use them.

Disinfection is the destruction of the disease germs in or on infected material, and a disinfectant is a substance or agent that destroys disease germs. As they are usually employed, the words "disinfectant" and "germicide" are synonymous. An antiseptic is a substance that prevents the growth of germs without necessarily destroying them.

There are two opposing forces in infection–the disease germ and the defensive force of the animal body. The ability of germs to invade depends primarily on the number present and their vigour. The healthy animal body is able to resist invasion by considerable numbers of germs, especially if the germs have lost most of their original vigour. On the other hand, an animal in poor condition is generally more susceptible to infection.

The essential sources of disease germs are the bodies of diseased animals. After leaving such animals, the germs die or tend to lose their vigour. Their survival outside the animal body is favoured by the presence of manure and other waste matter–the substances to which we give the general name "dirt."

The importance of cleanliness in the care of animals cannot be emphasized too much. Proper cleaning removes most of the germs along with the dirt that protects them, and the remaining germs are usually so weakened or so few in number that they are harmless under ordinary conditions.

If in addition to having clean surroundings the animals themselves are kept clean, well-fed, and in good condition, there is ordinarily no need for the use of disinfectants. If disease breaks out, however, it will be necessary to make use of disinfectants as well as of the usual cleaning agents. Since the sick animal is the original source of infection it should be kept away from healthy animals, and since the number and vigour of disease germs are greatest near their source in the sick animal the best place to use disinfectants is in its immediate vicinity. The materials to be disinfected include manure, urine, and other body discharges and bedding or other material soiled by such discharges. If infected material is scattered, it becomes necessary to apply disinfectants very extensively and thoroughly in order to be sure of reaching all of it.

In some instances–for example, in scabies–disease is caused by insect like parasites which are very small but not microscopic in size. In combating such diseases the destruction of the causative organism is usually accomplished through total immersion of the infected animal in a solution that is poisonous to the parasite but not dangerous to the animal. Such a process is called dipping, and the substance used for preparing the solution, or the solution itself, is called a dip. In cattle tick fever, formerly known as Texas fever, the causative organism is microscopic in size, but the disease is combated by destroying the tick that carries the micro-organism; hence in this case also dips are employed. A few chemicals or compounded mixtures may be useful for both dipping and disinfection, but there is no necessary relationship between dips and disinfectants because insects and ordinary disease germs are so different that a substance fatal to one may not be harmful to the other. Dips are therefore usually considered in a class by themselves, apart from disinfectants.

Disinfectants differ from one another in many of their properties, including their ability to kill micro-organisms, and germs also differ widely in their susceptibility to the various disinfectants. No single disinfectant is efficient against the germs of all diseases, nor is any disinfectant equally effective against the same germ under all conditions, for the activity of every disinfectant is influenced by such factors as the time of exposure to the disinfectant, temperature, chemical reaction and concentration, and the kind and amount of organic matter that may be present. Strictly speaking, there is no such thing as a "general disinfectant." So far as possible a disinfectant should be selected for its efficiency against the germs of a particular disease and its suitability for use in the place where it is to be applied.

General Rules for Using Disinfectants

No matter what disinfectant may be chosen, however, there are certain general principles to be considered in using it. In the first place, since very few disinfectants act instantaneously even under the most favourable circumstances, it, is always necessary to allow them ample time. In the second place, temperature has a great effect on the activity of disinfectants. Cold decreases and heat increases activity, so disinfecting solutions should, if possible, be used warm, or even hot. Furthermore, under practical conditions there is always more or less dirt present, especially manure and other organic materials. Most disinfectants penetrate slowly and poorly, especially when organic matter is present. Solutions usually penetrate better than emulsions, while gaseous disinfectants cannot be depended on to penetrate to any depth. If manure or other similar material is to be disinfected, it must be broken up and thoroughly mixed with the disinfecting solution so that the latter is distributed through the mass.

Since organic matter serves to protect disease germs and otherwise interferes with the activity of disinfectants, disinfection should always be preceded by thorough cleaning. All manure, bedding, and rubbish in stables or barnyards should be removed to a place inaccessible to livestock and burned, if possible, or thoroughly mixed with disinfectant. Then after the area has been cleaned with hot water and soap or washing soda, the disinfecting solution should be applied liberally and thoroughly. If only a small surface is to be disinfected, the solution may be applied with a whitewash brush. In all cases, however, the best method of application is by means of a spray pump.

Principal Disinfecting Agents and Substances

Although no attempt will be made here to enumerate all the agents or substances that may be used to kill disease germs, some of the most useful physical agents and chemical substances will be discussed briefly. Among the physical agencies are sunlight and heat. Direct sunlight is an active germicide, but its intensity is so variable and its disinfecting power so superficial that it cannot be considered a reliable disinfecting agent. Heat may be applied in various ways. The chemical substances include acids, alkalies, compounds of various metals, chlorine and iodine and their compounds, and the general group that includes alcohol, carbolic acid, and substances chemically related to them. Some of these, such as sulfur dioxide and formaldehyde, are used as gases. The rest are used in solutions, usually in water.

Various substances or compounds are recommended or used as disinfectants on account of their odour. There is no connection between odour and disinfecting value, and disinfectants should be chosen only on account of their known disinfecting value.

Although none of the disinfecting agents or substances described in this article is universally useful, some of the simplest and least expensive can usually be employed in place of expensive proprietary preparations. When they can be used, such simple processes as burning, baking, boiling, or steaming will usually be more effective than any chemical disinfectant. Except for disinfection against the germs of tuberculosis, lime and lye, which are cheap and readily available, will be found quite generally satisfactory.

Heat in Various Forms

Burning is a most useful way of applying heat wherever circumstances permit. For example, if the place to be disinfected contains a great deal of rubbish and articles of little value, burning will often be cheaper and easier than disinfection. Burning is also the most satisfactory method of disinfecting and disposing of small amounts of infected body discharges.

Dry heat is not so satisfactory as moist heat, since it lacks penetrating power and scorches fabrics, but it may occasionally be preferred. The ordinary household oven may be used for the purpose, and it should be heated sufficiently to brown cotton slightly (to about 320° F.). Objects to be disinfected should remain in the oven at this temperature for at least 1 hour. Moist heat is most often employed as boiling water or steam. Exposure to boiling water will destroy all ordinary disease germs, although it sometimes fails to kill the spores of such diseases as anthrax (splenic fever) or tetanus (lockjaw). Many disease germs are killed by moist heat at temperatures much below the boiling point of water as, for example, in the pasteurization of milk, and most of the ordinary disease germs are killed by boiling water in a very few moments. Boiling water may be used for the disinfection of fabrics of many kinds and of articles or implements made of materials that are not injured by boiling. In disinfecting objects made of iron or steel the addition of 1 percent of carbonate of soda to the water will prevent rusting. Although, as stated above, most of the ordinary disease germs are killed by boiling water very quickly, it is advisable in practice to allow at least 10 minutes exposure so that every particle of the material to be disinfected may be heated to the required temperature.

Steam under pressure is perhaps the most effective of all disinfecting agents, but under farm conditions steam would usually be employed at atmospheric pressure as "streaming" steam. This has the same basic disinfecting power as boiling water, since streaming steam and boiling water have the same temperature–100° C. (212° F.). In practice, however, such steam requires a longer time to bring all of the material to be disinfected to the required temperature, and it is advisable, therefore, to allow an exposure of half an hour to an hour. Steam is useful for the disinfection of many kinds of material, but it shrinks woolen fabrics and ruins leather, fur, skins of all kinds, rubber shoes, oil cloth, and articles containing glue or varnish. Disinfection with streaming steam does not require any apparatus except a boiler to supply the necessary steam and a hose or tube to carry it. Feed bags or other articles of similar material may be disinfected by being hung in any sort of small compartment and treated with steam. Such a structure need not be tight, for the steam escaping through the cracks serves to produce a circulation that aids penetration of the heat.

Sulfur Dioxide

Sulfur dioxide is the gas liberated by burning sulfur. Although commonly used in the past, it is little used at present because it is too destructive to fabrics, colours, and metals. It is not a very good germicide and is more useful for the destruction of insects and vermin than for disinfection.

Formaldehyde Gas and Solution

Formaldehyde is practically the only gas suitable for general application because it does not injure fabrics, colours, or metals. The gas is used rather than the solution (formalin) where the value of materials, such as hay or fodder, would be lessened by wetting. Under farm conditions, however, its use is often impracticable. Since the gas escapes readily through any openings, compartments to be disinfected must be tightly closed and all openings sealed during the period of disinfection. Formaldehyde gas is not effective at temperatures much below 65°F., and it is desirable that the air be moist.

In disinfecting small compartments, formaldehyde solution (formalin) may be sprayed into the compartment and allowed to evaporate. At least 10 ounces of the solution should be used for every 1,000 cubic feet of space. For rooms and large compartments the usual method of liberating the gas is by the action of potassium permanganate on formalin. Since some of the formalin is used up in the chemical reaction with the permanganate, it is necessary to use 20 ounces of formalin and 16 2/3 ounces of potassium permanganate for the disinfection of 1,000 cubic feet of space. The permanganate is placed in a wide-bottomed bucket or basin and the formalin poured over it. Since the reaction between the two substances liberates considerable heat, it is advisable to place the container on bricks or some other suitable material in order to prevent injury to the floor. As the action of formaldehyde gas is quite superficial, objects or materials to be disinfected should be spread out so as to offer the greatest possible surface to the action of the formaldehyde. After the formaldehyde gas has been liberated, the room or compartment should be kept tightly closed for at least 8 hours before it is opened and aired.

Formaldehyde solution is often used for disinfecting objects that are not injured by wetting. Its disinfecting power is great and not much affected by organic matter, but since it acts rather slowly ample, time must be allowed. Formalin does not injure metals except after prolonged action, and it does not injury ordinary fabrics. It is not suitable for disinfecting furs because it tends to harden skills and make them brittle. It is usually employed in a 10-percent solution in water.

Boric and Acetic Acids

Boric acid is a very feeble germicide, although it is often used in solution as an application for the eyes and other sensitive parts of the body. Acetic acid is a more effective germicide, and the amount usually found in full-strength vinegar (usually about 5 percent) is sufficient to kill some of the less resistant disease germs. It is a stronger acid than boric and too irritating for application to the eyes or other sensitive parts of the body. Vinegar is sometimes used in the treatment of local infections or of skin diseases.

Lime and Lye

Lime is a very cheap and useful disinfectant. It is usually employed in the form of "milk of lime." Only quicklime should be used, since air-slaked lime is practically useless. The quicklime is first slaked by adding 1 pint of water to 2 pounds of quicklime. Milk of lime is obtained by adding 4 parts of water to 1 of the slaked lime and mixing thoroughly. Whitewash may be prepared by adding water to milk of lime until a mixture of suitable density is obtained.

The following formulas for special whitewashes (from Farmers' Bulletin 1452, Painting on the Farm) may be found useful:

Whitewash No.1 (for sheds, etc.)

Carefully slake half a bushel (38 pounds) of good quicklime; strain the paste, while still thick, through wire fly screen and add it to a solution made by dissolving 15 pounds of common salt in 7½ gallons of water, mixing thoroughly. Thin with more water.

Whitewash No.2 (for sheds, etc.)

Carefully slake half a bushel (38 pounds) of good quicklime; strain the paste, while still thick, through wire fly screen and add about 4 gallons of hot water. While stirring vigourously pour into the lime mixture a solution made by first dissolving 12 pounds of salt and 6 ounces of alum in about 4 gallons of hot water and then adding 1 quart of molasses. Thin with water.

Whitewashing will help to make fences, pens, and outbuildings sanitary, besides improving their appearance. Milk of lime is well suited for use around dairy barns because it lacks odor. It is not effective, however, against the spores of germs that cause anthrax and lockjaw or against the germs of tuberculosis.

Ordinary lye usually contains about 94 percent of a chemical known as sodium hydroxide, which is a very effective disinfectant. It is effective against the viruses of foot-and-mouth disease and hog cholera and the germs of fowl cholera and bacillary white diarrhea of young chicks. In strong solutions it is effective against the spores of anthrax but not against the germs of tuberculosis. It is usually employed as a 2 per cent solution in water, but for disinfection against anthrax it is necessary to use a 5 per cent solution. A 2 per cent solution may be prepared by adding 1 pound of lye to 5½ gallons of water. In cases where lime is not objectionable, the addition of 2½ pounds of water-slaked (not air-slaked) lime to the 5½ gallons of lye solution to form a whitewash will increase the effectiveness of the solution by preventing the transformation of the sodium hydroxide into a carbonate.

A whitewash made in this way should not be applied to materials that are injured by lye. *Concentrated lye is a caustic poison. Care should be taken to avoid getting any of it into the eyes or breathing in any of the fine dust that may arise while handling the dry material. Solutions should be so disposed of as to prevent injury to livestock.* Solutions of lye are injurious to painted or varnished surfaces and to woolen or silk fabrics if allowed to remain in contact with them for a considerable period of lime. Since they do not injure bare wood, earthenware, enamelware, or any of the common metals except aluminum, they may be kept in containers made of these materials. Since exposure to the air soon converts sodium hydroxide to the relatively inactive sodium carbonate, containers should be kept tightly covered.

Various Chemical Compounds

Sodium carbonate and trisodium phosphate are used chiefly as cleansing agents, but they also have appreciable disinfecting value. If they are to be used in solution for disinfecting purposes at ordinary temperatures it is advisable to add 0.5 per cent of sodium hydroxide, but if the solutions are to be used hot this will not be necessary. Sodium carbonate is obtainable in the form of washing soda, soda crystals, and also as soda ash. Washing soda should be used in 6 per cent and soda ash in 2 per cent solution. Trisodium phosphate can be obtained as tribasic phosphate of soda, which should be used in a 2.5 per cent solution.

The various inorganic compounds of mercury, especially the bichloride (corrosive sublimate), are known to be powerful disinfectants. They are not suitable for farm use, however, on account of the danger to the farm family and to livestock as well as their relatively high cost. From time to time various compounds of copper, arsenic, or zinc have been recommended as germicides, but they all have relatively little germicidal value. Sulfate of copper (blue vitriol), however, is extremely effective against algae, and since algae often cause unpleasant odours or tastes in drinking water, copper sulfate is sometimes added to water to check or destroy their growth.

Chlorine gas as a disinfectant is almost exclusively used for the treatment of water supplies or sewage. Some of its compounds, however, are widely used for disinfection on the farm. Chlorinated lime is commonly known also as chloride of lime, or bleaching powder. Although it is a powerful disinfectant its potency is greatly reduced by contact with organic matter, so that when it is employed for disinfecting manure or body discharges it must be used in considerable quantities. Since it is often of uncertain strength, is injurious to metals, and has an odour that is readily taken up by milk, it is not a very practical disinfectant, especially for use around dairy barns. It is usually employed in a water solution containing about 6 ounces to the gallon, or 1 pound to 3 gallons.

Besides chlorinated lime certain other chlorine compounds are in more or less general use. The hypochlorites, usually sold in solution and under various proprietary names, have been used quite extensively to disinfect dairy equipment such as milk cans and bottles. In the concentrations usually employed they are effective when applied to clean surfaces, but their efficiency, like that of chlorinated lime, is largely reduced by organic matter. They will not sterilize dirty equipment, and their application to surfaces that are not thoroughly clean is entirely useless. Chlorinated lime and the hypochlorites are not effective against the germs of tuberculosis.

Iodine

Iodine in solution is extensively used for skin disinfection, and it remains the standard for this purpose although there are many proprietary preparations containing organic compounds of mercury or silver that are widely advertised. Tincture of iodine is the solution most generally employed. Although complete sterilization of the skin by any disinfectant is almost impossible, the application of tincture of iodine for treatment of superficial wounds or for preparing the site for an operation does serve to reduce the number of disease germs to a minimum. Since dirt interferes with the germicidal efficiency of iodine, the skin should be cleaned as well as possible before the solution is applied.

Alcohol

Grain alcohol has been used more or less as a disinfectant, and laboratory tests have shown that it is effective against the less resistant disease germs, such as those that cause typhoid fever. Absolute alcohol or solutions containing less than 50 percent of alcohol have comparatively little germicidal value. The most effective solutions are those containing about 70 percent of alcohol–the amount usually contained in "rubbing" alcohol.

Carbolic Acid and Cresol

The term "carbolic acid" has been rather loosely employed to designate a variety of substances that are chemically related but differ in their disinfecting properties. Although so-called carbolic acid has been widely used as a farm disinfectant, there is little to be said in its favour. It is generally uncertain in composition, and it has no advantages over other disinfectants that are readily available. The true carbolic acid (phenol) is not well suited for disinfection on a large scale because it is expensive and not as powerful as other disinfectants that cost less. It may be found useful, however, for disinfection on a small scale. Carbolic acid is not effective against the virus of hog cholera or the spores of anthrax, but it is very effective against most of the ordinary disease germs. It is most often used in a 5 per cent solution in water. Carbolic acid and other similar disinfectants are not suitable for use in refrigerators or compartments where food is stored or in dairy barns, because food products tend to take up these substances from the air and acquire a disagreeable taste and odour.

Commercial cresol is known under various names such as tricresol, cresylic acid, and liquid carbolic acid. It consists of a mixture of closely related chemical compounds, all of which are superior to pure carbolic acid in disinfecting value. Cresol is not readily soluble in water and is therefore most generally used in mixtures with soap. It may, however, be used in a water solution in the same way as pure carbolic acid. Since it is more powerful than the latter, a 2 per cent solution of cresol may be considered the equivalent of a 5 per cent solution of carbolic acid. Unlike carbolic acid, cresol is effective against the virus of hog cholera.

A soap solution of cresol, known as the compound solution of cresol, is described in the United States Pharmacopoeia (U.S.P. XI, Liquor Cresolis Saponatus) and may be obtained at drug stores. A substitute for the compound solution of cresol, known as saponified cresol (also called cresylic disinfectant) is sold by companies dealing in disinfectants. Saponified cresol is cheaper than the compound solution and is just as good a disinfectant. It is extensively used for disinfection under the supervision of the Bureau of Animal Industry. Saponified cresol is usually employed in a water solution, 4 ounces to a gallon of water. Solutions of cresol should not be used in or near compartments where food is kept, on account of the odour. Soap solutions of cresol do not mix well with hard water.

Besides disinfectants containing cresol in soap solution there are many proprietary disinfectants that contain cresol along with coal-tar oils and soap in mixtures that form milky emulsions in water. The disinfecting power of these products varies. Since there is no trustworthy method of determining their relative values by chemical analysis, they are compared by laboratory tests on typhoid fever germs. They are tested along with carbolic acid (phenol), and their values in comparison with it are expressed in the form of a "phenol coefficient." Since these coal-tar-emulsion disinfectants vary so much in disinfecting value, it is advisable to use only those that have a guaranteed phenol coefficient. However, since phenol coefficients are determined under laboratory conditions that are likely to differ from conditions in practical disinfection, the coefficient often does not accurately indicate the relative values of disinfectants in actual use. Thus it is safer to use these disinfectants, especially in the presence of organic matter, in concentrations twice as great as would be indicated by the phenol coefficient.

In the disinfection of dairy barns and similar places in the campaign for eradication of tuberculosis the cresol disinfectants have been found objectionable on account of their odour. Under such conditions a disinfectant called sodium orthophenylphenate is extensively used because it is free from objectionable odour.

Soaps

Soaps have some germicidal power, especially when used with hot water, but this power is rather limited. Cleaning with soap and hot water kills some of the less resistant disease germs but the effect is largely mechanical through the removal of dirt and infective material. Of the soaps commercially available those prepared exclusively from coconut oil, such as so-called salt-water soap, usually have the greater disinfecting value. Medicated soaps, in general, have little disinfecting power and cannot be relied upon to destroy resistant organisms.

Chapter 8

HOW RESEARCH AIDS IN DISEASE CONTROL

John R. Mohler[1]

[1] *John R. Mohler is Chief of the Bureau of Animal Industry.*

What are the problems of research in animal disease? How does research tackle these problems? What does it accomplish? How is it organized? These are the questions considered by the Chief of the Bureau of Animal Industry.

In the United States Department of Agriculture and cooperating agricultural institutions, groups of skilled scientific workers have been assembled to whom not only agricultural interests but a number of others as well look for the solution of many perplexing problems (*1*).[2] These problems run the gamut of human experience, but most of the questions, now as in the past, are concerned with improving man's security from the dangers that beset him and his means of livelihood. Adequate food, clothing, and shelter are still the basic needs. In their attainment, domestic animals have long been utilized.

Development of Veterinary Science

Man early learned to guard his domestic animals from wild beasts, but he has had much greater difficulty in dealing with enemies of microscopic size that cause diseases. That the contagious nature

[1] Italic numbers in parentheses refer to Literature Cited.

of several animal diseases was recognized as early as the first century is clearly indicated in the writings of Columella, whose observations on animal and human health caused him to urge the segregation of the sick as a means of preventing the spread of infection.

Early in the Christian Era, Vegetius, another Roman writer, urged a revival of interest in what was then known as veterinary art, in order to curb losses from outbreaks of animal plagues. Much later, about the time of Galileo, modern science, and with it the methods known today as those of scientific research, began to develop. Facilities for research in disease were meager, however, until the development of the microscope by the Dutch naturalist, Leeuwenhoek, in the seventeenth century. Since then, and particularly since the discoveries of Pasteur, veterinary science has been marked by a succession of discoveries that have greatly reduced hazards to animal life. Throughout the world diligent scientific workers have traced scores of animal diseases to their sources, revealing as causes specific viruses, bacteria, parasites, toxins, and nutritive deficiencies.

During the period from 1860 to 1885 the names of foreign scientists, including Pasteur, Koch, Lister, and Davaine, dominated veterinary literature. But soon after the establishment of the United States Bureau of Animal Industry by Congress in 1884, Salmon and Smith (7), of the United States, laid the foundation of bacterin therapy-the use of bacterial extracts for disease prevention–and since then veterinary science in this country has commanded worldwide respect and recognition.

Scientific research is inherently altruistic. It has no local, regional, or national boundaries and knows no barriers of race or creed. Any professional lines of separation or demarcation are purely artificial, for research deals essentially with the collection of facts and the operation of natural laws that embrace all science. Veterinary research is based primarily on a group of fundamental sciences–biology, pathology, and parasitology–but it includes many others, such as chemistry, serology, and immunology. Statistical analyses of data have also been used with increasing frequency in recent years. Although great discoveries are occasionally accidental, the vast majority are the result of planning, patience, and critical evaluation of experimental findings.

It is regrettable that technical terminology has tended to act as a barrier to a better public understanding of research studies and services. There is, however, nothing inherently formidable about scientific terms. Like mechanical terms such as "carburetor" and "differential," many of them gradually become a part of common speech. One purpose of this article is to remove the aura of magic and mystery that often surrounds research and to show its intensely practical nature and its value to agriculture and industry.

A Typical Research Problem and its Solution

A brief account of the development of a typical research project will serve to illustrate the definite manner in which science contributes to livestock health.

A certain stunted condition and rather high death losses among young pigs were reported by large numbers of swine growers in the Middle West some years ago. When cases were investigated by a field veterinarian, they were usually described by the owners about as follows: "My sows farrowed good litters of healthy pigs. They were doing fine until several weeks old. Then they stopped growing and began coughing, 'thumping,' and dying."

Post mortem examination of pigs from such farms revealed the presence of ascarid (roundworm) larvae in the windpipe and lungs. Observation of the surroundings showed that where these troubles occurred the pigs were housed and fed on lots where hogs had been kept continuously for many years. Associated with such conditions were cases of intestinal inflammation, sore mouth, and lungworm infestation.

The next step taken by the investigators was an intensive study of the life cycle of the swine ascarid, a history that proved to be highly involved. One key to the problem had been provided by F.H. Stewart, a medical officer of the British Army stationed in Hong Kong, who had studied the ascarid of man and found that it followed a circuitous route in the human body. The swine ascarid also was soon found to follow a devious route through the pig, including visits to most of the vital organs and a brief stay in the windpipe and lungs. The last explained the coughing and the thumping noises in the chest.

The study also involved the determination of conditions that would limit the development of ascarid eggs, their resistance to chemicals, heat, and cold, and their longevity under various circumstances. A thorough examination of all scientific literature having a direct or indirect bearing on the problem was also made. All these lines of research were directed by B.H. Ransom, at that time chief of the Bureau's Zoological Division.

Investigators assigned to the problem found live embryos in ascarid eggs that had been buried as long as 375 days in soil in northern Illinois, where winters are severe and summers hot. Infected soil would thus remain dangerous for long periods. From all available data bearing on the problem, Ransom concluded that the key to the health and normal development of newly farrowed pigs was to protect them from infection with worm eggs. "It would seem," he, stated, "that the chief source of infection in the case of young pigs is the dirt-soiled skin of the sow." He therefore advised the thorough cleaning of farrowing quarters with lye solution and the brushing of all loose litter and mud from the sides of sows before they farrowed. He proposed that the sows' udders especially should be washed with soap and water and that the sows be placed in clean farrowing pens several days before the litters were expected.

Besides specifying clean conditions at the birth of the pigs, his plan provided also for keeping the young pigs on clean pasture, to which the sows and litters would be hauled, not driven, so as to prevent any contact with the soil.

After being placed on the clean pasture, the young pigs, of course, would sooner or later be exposed to the danger of swallowing some roundworm eggs passed by the sow, but the chances of infection, at any rate of heavy infestation, from this source when the eggs were scattered over a large, clean pasture, were considered to be relatively small by Ransom and his associates.

This general plan, based on research findings, was revolutionary in swine production. It proposed to change long-established practices in hog raising. It took pigs from their usual dusty lots or muddy wallows and put them in a pasture "parlour." At first swine growers were inclined to be skeptical of the new method. They awaited practical tests with interest. The system had its first trial under farm conditions in the fall of 1919 in McLean County, Ill. (*8*). This county was chosen because of the large previous losses there and assurances of cooperation from members of the local farm bureau. The first year 17 farmers agreed to cooperate in the project; later others joined until the total number of cooperators was 34.

Records of the results were kept for a period of 6 years. During that time 6,204 sows farrowed 47,536 pigs, of which 39,855 were placed on pasture. When losses from all causes were included, 76 percent of all the pigs farrowed were marketed and 24 percent were lost. Records showed that the losses were from stillbirths, accidents in farrowing and on pasture, hog cholera, worms, and all other diseases. Under ordinary farm conditions with pigs in old hog lots, about 50 percent of the pigs farrowed are normally marketed. Thus, under the sanitation system, 6 pigs were marketed to 2 lost, whereas under ordinary conditions 4 would have been marketed and 4 lost. On this basis, under the sanitation system the farmer can raise more pigs with the same number of sows, or he can raise as many but better pigs with fewer sows. In either case he can get a larger return for the feed consumed.

Further study of the experimental data showed that the system was much more effective in attaining the purpose for which it was intended than the foregoing results indicate. A system designed to control parasites should not be expected to protect pigs from hog cholera, stillbirth, and miscellaneous accidents. When such losses were excluded and the sanitation system was judged solely for its ability to control parasites and related filth-borne diseases, the records showed it to be nearly 98 percent effective. As was to be expected, some cooperators followed the various steps in the system more faithfully than others. Those whose cooperation was only fair obtained about 94 percent efficiency in preventing parasites and filth-borne diseases, whereas those following the system to the letter attained almost 99 percent.

The foregoing example illustrates the manner in which research is conducted and applied. Notwithstanding the seemingly revolutionary nature of the practice of taking sows out of old hog lots and washing them, the system has been widely adopted by hog raisers in all parts of the country, and they have obtained results substantially the same as those recorded in the field trials described. (See Fig. 1.) A modified form of the swine-sanitation system to combat kidney worms of swine in the South has likewise proved highly effective (9).

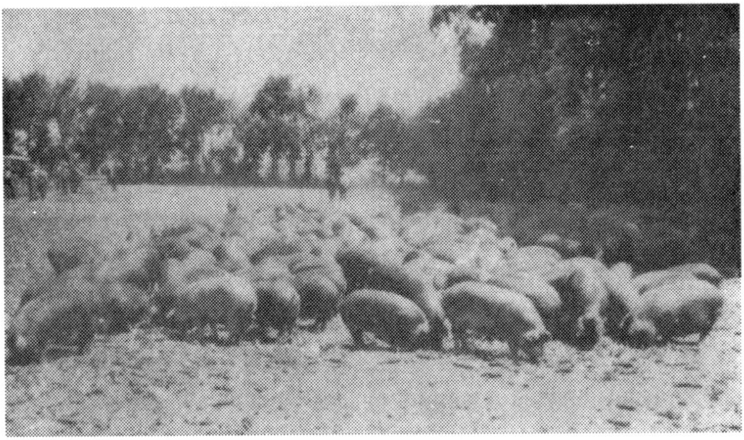

Fig. 1: A practical result of veterinary research—a uniformly healthy and well-grown lots of pigs raised free of parasites in accordance with sanitary methods.

Recent Advances in Veterinary Science Through Research

Much of the Department's scientific work has been developed in this way, to meet pressing needs, to throw up defenses quickly against pests, and to solve economic problems; yet at the same time it has added to knowledge of basic laws and principles. In the veterinary field the more notable discoveries and their application may be summarized as follows:

The principle that injection of sterilized cultures or dead bacteria confers immunity to subsequent inoculation with virulent material.

Simultaneous injection of immune serum and virulent blood as a means of immunization.

Proof that certain diseases can be carried from one animal to another only by an intermediate insect host.

Discovery of the nature of cattle tick fever, leading to a successful method of eradicating cattle ticks.

Development of a method of testing the strength of dips in vats.

Discovery that hog cholera is caused by a filtrable virus, and the development of a product that produces lasting immunity.

Development of crystal-violet vaccine against hog cholera.

Discovery and perfection of a practical, rapid method of tattooing hogs, which has been especially useful in determining the original ownership of hogs shipped to market.

Perfection of a serological method–that is, one based on the reaction of blood serum in a laboratory test–of diagnosing the disease dourine.

Success in destroying trichinae in pork by refrigeration.

Development of a Federal meat-inspection service, based on scientific principles, that has won world-wide recognition.

Discovery of a new and effective remedy for hookworms in dogs that has also been used successfully on millions of human beings infected with hookworms.

Development of methods of preventing losses from roundworms and kidney worms of swine.

Improvement in methods of making tuberculin, used in tuberculosis eradication.

Discovery of a rapid, stained-antigen test, highly useful in the detection and eradication of pullorum disease in poultry.

Development of numerous effective dips and disinfectants.

Discovery of phenothiazine as an effective anthelmintic, or worm medicine.

Successful use of barium antimonyl tartrate to remove gapeworms from chickens.

Improvement in the diagnosis and treatment of bovine mastitis.

Investigation of brucellosis (Bang's disease), leading to successful calfhood vaccination.

Development of a vaccine to combat encephalomyelitis.

Improvement in methods of handling livestock and livestock products in interstate and foreign trade.

Advancement in standards of veterinary education and of private practice, including hospitalization and the use of biological products, anesthetics, and the X-ray.

Coincident with the advances in veterinary science just mentioned, research workers have made extensive contributions to modern knowledge of livestock breeding, feeding, management, housing, and sanitation.

Research in Relation to Regulatory Measures

A very close relation exists between research findings and regulatory measures designed for the protection of animals and the whole-someness of their products. Scientific knowledge enables veterinary officials, for instance, to determine the feasibility of regulatory measures for accomplishing a specified purpose. The practical eradication of bovine tuberculosis from the United States is based on knowledge concerning the cause and spread of the disease and the dependability of the tuberculin test as a means of diagnosis (*10*). Systems of meat and milk inspection have their foundation in the bedrock of scientific knowledge. The selection and use of the proper dips and disinfectants for combating animal diseases depend on thoroughgoing tests of various chemicals.

Since successful law enforcement is based to a considerable degree on the testimony of expert witnesses, in branches of public service that operate under the direction of regulatory officials there is need for experts qualified in various fields of science.

Veterinary Research Helps Protect Human Health

As previously pointed out, research in veterinary science has had numerous applications in human medicine. The constant operation of the Federal meat-inspection service (*4*) in approximately 700 establishments throughout the United States is a further means of protecting human health. In the course of their work, inspectors have to be on the watch for no less than 50 diseases and conditions for which condemnations of animal carcasses are made. Of these, have been found to be transmissible to man through fresh meat–tuberculosis, anthrax, glanders, trichinosis, brucellosis (in man usually called undulant fever), and a tapeworm infestation known scientifically as cysticercosis. Knowledge provided by research concerning these and other diseases has established means by which man may protect himself from infections that might otherwise be dangerous or even fatal.

A useful aid to human health, developed within the last half century, is the preparation of extracts from the glands of animals slaughtered in inspected packing establishments. Medical science has shown that deficiencies in the glands of human beings may be corrected by the skillful use of preparations from those of healthy animals. Since many of the glands are small–for example, the pituitary, parathyroid, and suprarenal–several thousand of them are sometimes necessary to make as much as a pound of finished extract. Large-scale slaughtering operations, combined with thorough veterinary inspection, are accordingly necessary as a basis for this branch of the pharmaceutical industry. A high degree of technical skill based on extensive research is, of course, necessary in the preparation and standardization of the hundred or more glandular extracts that are made commercially for medical use.

Occasionally the relationship between animal and human health is highly involved, and the means by which the offending organism gains entrance to a vulnerable part of the body may even seem fantastic. One of the tapeworms, *Diphyllobothrium latum*, has a life cycle which involves temporary residence in a carnivore, such as a dog or cat, then in a crustacean, next in a fresh-water fish, and finally in a human being, in whose intestine the tapeworm mal grow to a length of 25 feet or more. Each stage of the tapeworm's development must be in the host specified in the order given. Any break in the cycle destroys the parasite. Man's simplest positive protection against this tapeworm, then, is to cook fish thoroughly.

In the case of anthrax (3), a disease affecting cattle and some other species, research has disclosed the danger to livestock owners who fail to curb their natural tendency to open a carcass. The anthrax organism is extremely virulent, frequently having fatal effects. The body fluids of an animal dead of anthrax teem with the bacilli, and a post-mortem examination with the bare hands invites fatal infection. In its literature the Department of Agriculture is emphatic in warning against this danger. Research has also disclosed the danger to man from other animal diseases, among which rabies, or hydrophobia, is especially serious (5). Fortunately the Pasteur treatment prevents death from hydrophobia.

In conducting their investigations, research workers often undergo exposure to organisms that are either known to be dangerous to human life or are proved to be so as the studies develop. Many workers have suffered impaired health, and some have died as martyrs of public service. Zealous, public-spirited scientists have at times also used themselves as subjects of tests for which laboratory animals were deemed unsuitable.

Results of Research Available to All

In keeping with the basic policy of the United States Department of Agriculture to gather and disseminate useful information, the results of research are promptly made available to scientific organizations and to the public.

Although scientific knowledge is utilized in some of its aspects chiefly by professional workers, it is equally available to interested laymen and others concerned. This broad policy is desirable because the further advancement of science depends on public interest and understanding, because the diffusion of knowledge is a fundamental principle of a democracy, and because it enables producers who are not themselves scientists to use scientific principles in their work-in fact they must use them to be successful under modern conditions.

In the research field, as in industry, many discoveries constitute improvements or refinements in methods. For instance, tuberculin, employed in the test for the presence of tuberculosis, has been known and used for many years, but the present type of tuberculin is a greatly improved product as compared with that first made and used by its originator, Koch. The present improved, or so-called new, tuberculin is grown on a synthetic medium of controlled composition and is about 10 percent more efficient than the former type.

Cooperation of Research Workers with Livestock Owners

The research worker in veterinary science is far from being a recluse, as he is so often pictured. More often he carries on his work in cooperation with other technically trained associates and tests the practical application of his findings to a considerable extent with farmers on their own farms. This was the procedure used in the development of the swine-sanitation system, described earlier in this article.

Another example was the conduct of research on hog cholera that led to the preventive-serum treatment. During the period 1897-1907 three Department investigators, Marion Dorset, C.N. McBryde, and W. B. Niles (Fig. 2), conducted a series of experiments on hog cholera in southwestern Iowa, near Sidney (2). The disease had been

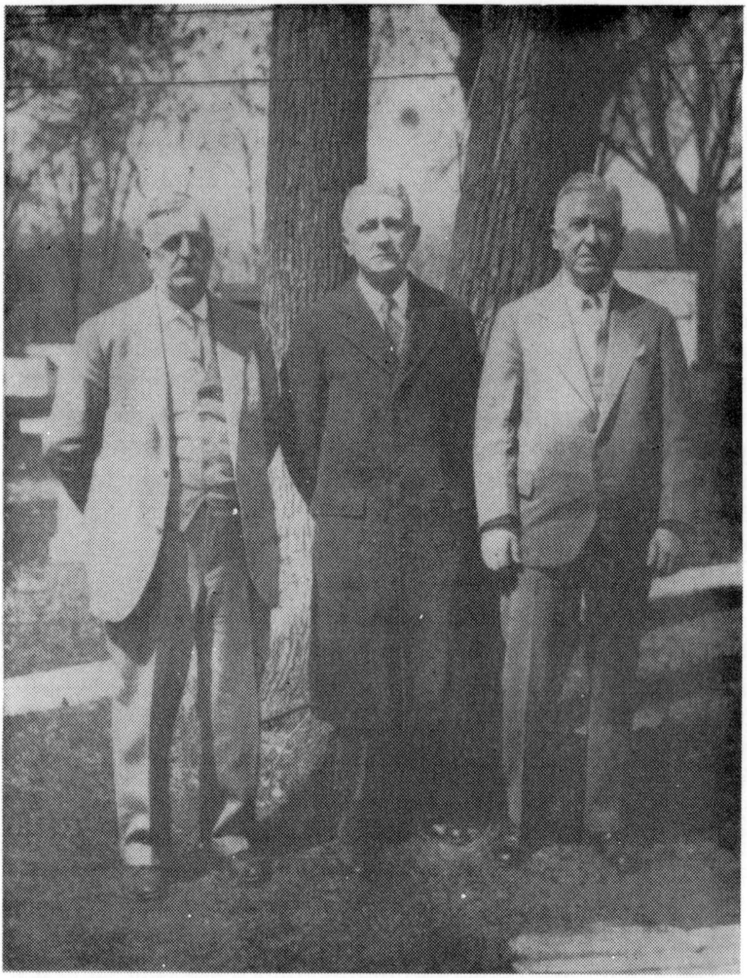

Fig. 2: The discoverers of anti-hog-cholera serum. Left to right, W.B. Niles, Marion Dorset, and C.N. McBryde. This picture was taken at the scene of their first experiments, near Sidney, Iowa.

causing serious losses there, and samples of disease-producing blood from natural outbreaks were thus readily obtainable. After many technical studies these workers finally developed a serum that gave promising results on a small laboratory scale. They then sought and obtained the cooperation of swine owners in making tests under practical farm conditions.

Figure 3, a photograph of one of the early cooperators, J.K. Peterson, is of historical interest.

Before the discovery of this method of immunization, entire herds of hogs often fell victim to cholera about the time they were ready for market. Today the inexpensive, practical serum treatment is a positive protection against such losses. The process is made available to all persons by a public-service patent, and still further protection is provided through Federal legislation for assuring serum of satisfactory purity and potency. Since the original discovery, continued research has resulted in improvement of serum by clarifying, concentrating, and pasteurizing processes.

In dealing with other disease problems, also, research workers have maintained close association with practical farmers, veterinarians, and others concerned in the use of preventive or control measures. The development and testing of the vaccine used

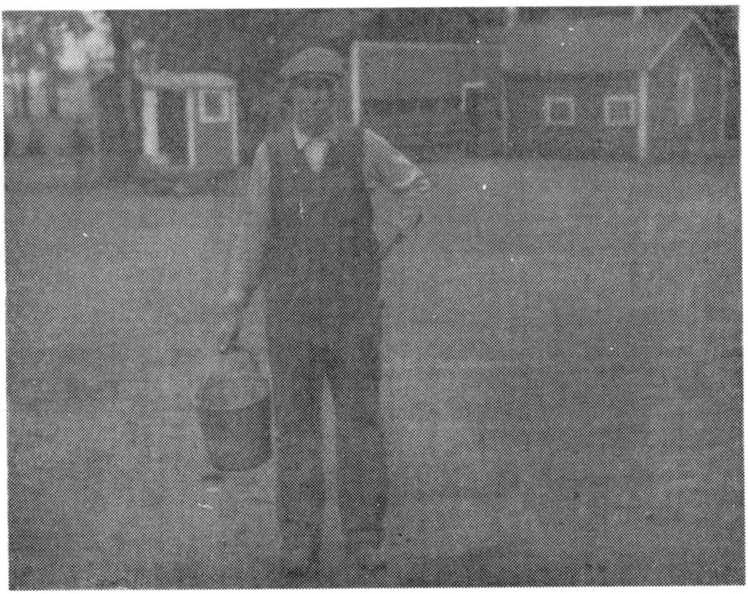

Fig. 3: J.K. Peterson, a farmer-cooperator, whose herd of hogs was one of the first to be immunized with anti-hog-cholera serum.

in calfhood vaccination for the prevention of brucellosis (6) involved field trials on more than 260 herds in 24 States before the Bureau of Animal Industry considered the vaccine sufficiently perfected for general use.

Simplicity in the treatment of disease is naturally desired by most livestock owners, and research is directed to that end. Yet the nature of animal maladies is such that the best method of prevention or control varies greatly in different diseases. In one case it may be a vaccine, in another a serum, in still another a chemical dip, and is dealing with internal parasites it may be an anthelmintic. In controlling tuberculosis, brucellosis, and pullorum disease the usual procedure is to apply a diagnostic test and dispose of the animals that prove by a positive reaction to have the disease.

Various complexities may enter disease situations so that the goal of simplicity cannot be attained. One of the newer means of disease control, which has been successful in treating trichomoniasis of the lower digestive tract of turkeys–a disease easily confused with blackhead–is the artificial elevation of temperature, so-called fever therapy. Exposure of birds in a cabinet (Fig. 4) where the temperature is about 104°F. and the relative humidity about 65 percent results in an internal temperature in the body 2° to 6° above normal, which in turkeys is 106.5° F. Several of these heat treatments, lasting from 1 to 2 hours each, have resulted in early improvement and a large percentage of cures.

With all the skill and ingenuity of research workers in solving disease problems, the fact remains that, in most cases, simple cleanliness, combined with care to exclude infection from the premises, is the best and cheapest insurance of livestock health. For the greatest success with this method; however, buildings and equipment should be designed and constructed so that sanitary standards can be effectively maintained. Figure 5 illustrates an insanitary environment in which an entire flock of poultry was lost from the inroads of bronchitis. In general, sanitation may be considered the first line of defense, with veterinary science and services backing it up.

Congressional Control Over Federal Research

As a control over the kind, amount, and cost of research conducted by the Department of Agriculture, congressional

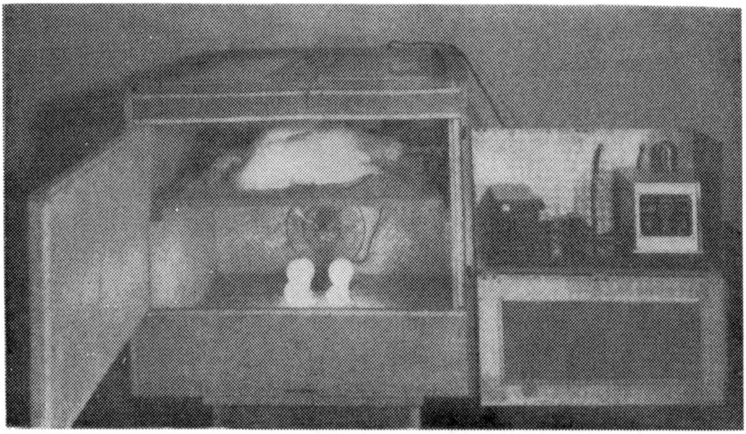

Fig. 4: Treating trichomoniasis in a turkey by fever therapy. The temperature of the cabinet is carefully controlled thermostatically.

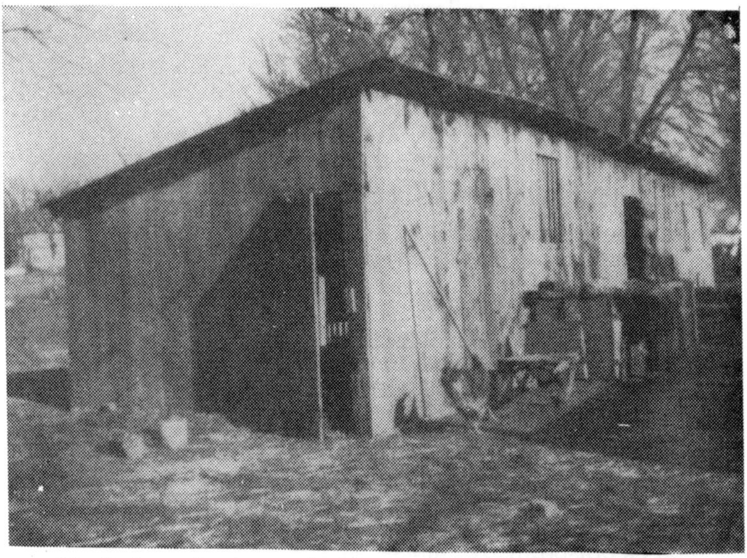

Fig. 5: A poultry house lacking proper light and ventilation. An outbreak of infectious bronchitis among chickens housed in this structure was so severe that disposal of the entire flock was necessary.

committees for many years have weighed the merits of various projects proposed by research leaders. After full consideration of the available facts and prospective benefits in each case, Congress authorizes only those projects that are deemed to be in the best public interest. Thus the people of the United States, under the authority vested in their congressional representatives, have a controlling hand over the services that research workers seek to render.

From time to time special legislative acts have authorized the establishment and support of regional and other experiment stations. The Bankhead-Jones law, for instance, in 1935 provided for basic research of specified kinds in the Department of Agriculture and in the State experiment stations and land-grant colleges. This law directed the Secretary of Agriculture to conduct research for improving the quality of agricultural commodities, to discover uses for farm products and byproducts, and to study the conservation, development, and use of land.

Animal diseases being studied by the Bureau of Animal Industry under current projects, following authorization by Congress, include the following:

Brucellosis of cattle.

Mastitis of cattle.

Tuberculosis.

Paratuberculosis (Johne's disease).

Nutritional deficiencies of cattle.

Bovine trichomoniasis.

Calf scours.

Anaplasmosis of cattle.

Equine encephalomyelitis and forage poisoning.

Rabies.

Swine erysipelas.

Swine influenza.

Miscellaneous diseases, including blackleg, paratyphoid infection of swine, foot rot, and alkali disease.

Stock poisoning by plants.

Poultry diseases, including laryngotracheitis, fowl paralysis, tuberculosis, pullorum disease, and fowl pox.

Methods of producing immunization against hog cholera.

Periodic ophthalmia of equines.

Parasitic diseases of animals, including parasites of livestock, dogs, cats, and wild animals.

Mechanisms of infection in contagious, infectious, and parasitic diseases of domestic animals and poultry and methods of control.

To cope with many of the foregoing diseases on their home grounds, so to speak, the United States Bureau of Animal Industry maintains field stations in various parts of the country. The principal ones devoted to veterinary studies are:

The Animal Disease Station, Beltsville, Md., the staff of which collaborates on specific problems with field cooperators in 7 States.

The Regional Poultry Research Laboratory, East Lansing, Mich., the staff of which cooperates with workers of 25 State experiment stations.

The Field Station, Ames, Iowa.

The Regional Animal Disease Research Laboratory, Auburn, Ala., the staff of which cooperates with workers of 13 Southern States.

Additional resources for the study of disease problems, usually of a regional nature, are provided by the assignment of trained men to work with State and local authorities and also to conduct laboratory studies of disease in connection with Federal meat inspection. Work of these types is conducted in Colorado, Georgia, Illinois, Kansas, Nebraska, New Mexico, Texas, and Utah. The studies frequently involve cooperation with additional States having related problems.

Research As a Humane Influence

Besides providing accurate information of a positive, useful nature, veterinary research has also shown the fallacy of many old beliefs. To a large degree science has caused the discontinuance of ineffective and often cruel treatments. It has shown that alleged diseases, such as "hollow horn," were purely imaginary; the hollow condition of cows' horns is entirely normal, and the old, cruel practice of drilling a hole in a horn and pouring in turpentine has largely disappeared. Research has been and will continue to be a powerful influence in alleviating animal suffering, partly by discouraging futile, barbarous methods of treatment, but principally by removing the causes of maladies. In conquering sheep scab, caused by a mite that burrows into the flesh, science has saved millions of sheep from the torments of these parasites.

Limitations of Proprietary Drugs

As a result of claims of manufacturers of proprietary products, livestock owners have spent large amounts of money for drugs. No drug remedy known to science will prevent or cure certain diseases, including hog cholera, infectious abortion of cattle, and blackhead of turkeys. (By drugs, of course, are not meant biological products, such as vaccines and bacterins, used to prevent or cure diseases.) Some manufacturers have claimed to have drugs or chemicals that will combat those maladies successfully; others claim for their drugs the ability to increase the milk yields of cattle and egg yields of fowls. Some claims have led credulous farmers to believe that the remedies will do things which no medicines will or can do. Dependable figures on the money spent annually for proprietary remedies are lacking, but conservative estimates indicate that it considerably exceeds 10 million dollars. Some dairymen with meager incomes have spent as much as $10 a pound for worthless abortion remedies. A survey by the Federal Food and Drug Administration embracing the field of veterinary preparations disclosed more than 1,000 misbranded or worthless antiseptics, stock powders, liniments, salves, and similar products. Broadly speaking, the investment in such questionable articles would have yielded vastly better results in improved health of livestock if the money had been expended to improve sanitation and for capable veterinary services.

Veterinary Education

Fundamental training is, of course, necessary for the successful practice of veterinary medicine. It is likewise necessary for research work and related duties, including regulatory and administrative activities.

The chief sources of such training are the veterinary colleges maintained in conjunction with State universities and agricultural colleges. At the close of the fiscal year 1941 there were 10 of these veterinary institutions in the United States with equipment, faculties, and curricula affording 4 years or more of intensive study. As a means of safeguarding the quality of veterinary service, all the States and the District of Columbia have laws that regulate the practice of veterinary medicine. This form of supervision consists principally in licensing only properly trained and otherwise qualified and competent persons.

Research As a Public Service

A summary of the manner in which research aids in disease control and renders a broad public service properly includes the following observations:

In contrast to the fragmentary and inaccurate knowledge of a century ago concerning animal diseases, modern veterinary science provides dependable protection to the health of livestock.

Research is a fact-finding process that determines the soundness of previous beliefs or new hypotheses.

Research is altruistic, leading usually to the prompt announcement of results for use by any person anywhere.

As conducted in the United States, veterinary research is sponsored largely by the United States Department of Agriculture, agricultural experiment stations, and cooperating institutions.

For the most part, veterinary research is directed toward the solution of specific disease problems that have baffled livestock owners and on which they desire assistance. Research planned and conducted by trained specialists is the best known means of solving such problems.

More dependable knowledge concerning the nature and control of animal diseases has been assembled in the last 100 years than in all previous time.

Research is the foundation for the successful administration of animal quarantines, inspection services, and other beneficial regulations.

The results of research have alleviated suffering among the lower animals and greatly reduced the economic losses formerly caused by diseases, parasites, and related causes.

The net result of all types of veterinary service has been to surround the production of livestock and related food industries with increasingly effective safeguards. Discoveries in the course of such research have had many beneficial applications in other fields, including the advancement of human medicine.

Literature Cited

(1) CHEW, ARTHUR P. (1933). SCIENCE SERVING AGRICULTURE. U.S. Dept. Agr. Spec. Pub., 42 pp., illus.

(2) DORSET, M., McBRYDE, C.N., and NILES, W.B. (1908). FURTHER EXPERIMENTS CONCERNING THE PRODUCTION OF IMMUNITY FROM HOG CHOLERA. U.S. Bur. Anim. Indus. Bul. 102, 96 pp.

(3) GOCHENOUR, W. S. (1934). ANTHRAX. U.S. Dept. Agr. Farmers' Bul. 1736, 14 pp., illus.

(4) JOSS, EDWARD C. (1939). UNITED STATES MEAT INSPECTION. U. S. Dept. Agr. Yearbook (Food and Life) 1939: 355-359, illus.

(5) MOHLER, JOHN R. (1911). RABIES OR HYDROPHOBIA. U. S. Dept. Agr. Farmers' Bul. 449, 23 pp. (Revised 1923.)

(6) ________WIGHT, A.E., and O'REAR, H.M. (1941). CALFHOOD VACCINATION AS AN AID IN COOPERATIVE BANG'S DISEASE (BOVINE BRUCELLOSIS) CONTROL. Amer. Vet. Med. Assoc. Jour. 98: 1-9, illus.

(7) POWELL, FRED WILBUR. (1927). THE BUREAU OF ANIMAL INDUSTRY. ITS HISTORY, ACTIVITIES AND ORGANIZATION. Inst. Govt. Res., Serv. Monog. U.S. Govt., No. 47, 121 pp. Baltimore.

(8) RAFFENSPERGER, H.B., and CONNELLY, J.W. (1927). THE SWINE SANITATION SYSTEM AS DEVELOPED BY THE BUREAU OF ANIMAL INDUSTRY IN M'LEAN COUNTY, ILL. U.S. Dept. Agr. Tech. Bul. 44, 20 pp.

(9) SCHWARTZ, BENJAMIN (1934). CONTROLLING KIDNEY WORM IN SWINE IN THE SOUTHERN STATES. U.S. Dept. Agr. Leaflet 108, 6 pp., illus.

(10) WIGHT, ALEXANDER E. (1933). TUBERCULOSIS IN LIVESTOCK. DETECTION, CONTROL, AND ERADICATION. U.S. Farmers' Bul. 1069, 18 pp., illus.

Chapter 9

ORIGIN AND SPREAD OF IMPORTANT INSECT PESTS OF ANIMALS

H.H. Stage & J.A. Hyslop[1]

[1] *H.H. Stage is Senior Entomologist, Division of Insects Affecting Man and Animals, and J.A. Hyslop is Principal Entomologist, Division of Insect Pest Survey and Information, Bureau of Entomology and Plant Quarantine.*

A good many ages ago, insects originated the idea of thumbing a ride from one part of the country or one part of the world to another. Any conveyance suits them–an animal, bale of hay, a ship, automobile, or airplane, or just the winds that scud over land and sea. Here is a small part of the story of the world's craftiest and most dangerous stowaways.

As far back as the days of Pliny in the first century, and probably long before horses, cows, sheep, goats, dogs, and chickens were known to be infested with fleas, bots, and lice. Until the white man arrived in America not one of these animals had been present on this continent for a long time, with the possible exception of the dog. It is natural to assume therefore that all of the specific parasites that take so large an annual toll of our domestic animals were brought to the Western Hemisphere along with their hosts.

In the geological past, long before even the most remote historical periods, the American Continent was well supplied with ungulates, or hoofed animals. A great many species of wild horses were well established over much of the country, and elephants and camels were then indigenous. The hoofed animals disappeared during the early Quaternary geological period, estimated at a million years ago. The stony records of paleontology disclose a remarkable and interesting coincidence. In the Oligocene period some 40 million years ago, great shale beds were laid down in the vicinity of Florissant, Colo. These beds are particularly rich in insect fossils and have been very well explored. Among the fossilized insects is none other than a tsetse fly (Fig. 1), closely related to the fly that has practically prohibited the establishment of domestic animals in extensive areas of Africa. It is not impossible that this fly was the cause of the absolute extinction of the North American hoofed animals that might have carried the pests and parasites now found on domestic animals throughout the world. Because of the long lapse of time, however, between the early Quaternary period and the discovery North America, none of the lice, fleas, ticks, bots, and mites that now infest our domestic animals could have been on this

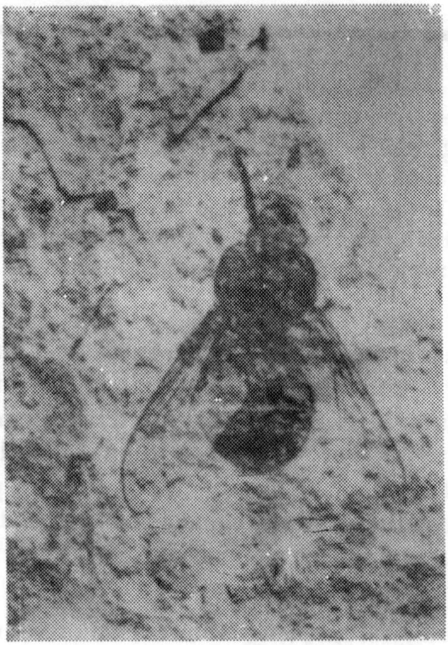

Fig. 1: A fossil tsetse fly.

continent when the early settlers arrived. Some of our domestic-animal pests do attack wild animals, but in most instances this is probably an adaptation of the pests to a different host. In a few instances, also, the natural enemies of wild animals have turned their attention to our domestic livestock.

In the early days many of the pests of plants were prevented from reaching this continent by the long period of overseas travel required and the lack of suitable food and habitat in transit. The pests of domestic animals, on the other hand, found a ship's hold full of their natural host animals an excellent place in which to live and reproduce; in fact, ship's holds often became unbearably infested with vermin.

Early breeders in North America were constantly seeking new sources of breeding stock. Not satisfied with the domestic cattle of Europe, they went farther and brought in the humped cattle (or zebu) from southeastern Asia, the Arabian horse, the peculiar varieties of poultry developed in India and China, the remarkable fur-bearing sheep of southwestern Asia, the Siamese cat, and the Pekingese dog. And all these introduced animals brought with them their peculiar pests and parasites.

Damage Done By Various Insect Pests

The insect pests of livestock are extremely important from an economic standpoint. It has been estimated that the damage to livestock amounts to $168,900,000 annually, and this does not include the loss occasioned by mosquitoes, horseflies, scab mites, and a large number of less important pests, or damage to animal products such as woolen goods and leather.

It may be illuminating to review the damage done by some of the pests already introduced into the country.

The northern cattle grub, *Hypoderma bovis*, first recorded here in 1910, is probably of European origin. It and a native species cause severe damage to hides and losses in beef and milk production amounting to over $65,000,000 annually.

Another insect, the nose botfly (*Gasterophilus haemorrhoidalis*) has been a serious pest of horses since it was first reported in this country. The early history of the occurrence of this insect in the United States seems to be somewhat clouded, but the earliest reports show that it was present in western North Dakota in 1883, in Montana in

1890, in Wyoming and Minnesota in 1910, in Nebraska in 1911, in Iowa in 1912, and in other States more recently. Just why this pest of horses did not become prominent years before these dates is difficult to tell. It seems almost certain that it was brought into this country at an early date with shipments of horses from Europe. The habits of the insect indicate that its dissemination is largely brought about by the movement of horses from place to place. The long time which the larvae spend within the host and the rather extended period during which they normally live away from the animal add to the danger of spread whenever horses are shipped or driven from infested to uninfested areas. Its failure to become established earlier may have been due to conditions surrounding the imported animals after arrival here, such as adverse climate. It is possible that climate may have a marked influence on the perpetuation of the species in any region and that it will not thrive in the more humid area east of the present area of great abundance, in North and South Dakota. Certainly it has become established in the United States only comparatively recently.

Another familiar pest is the sheep botfly (*Oestris ovis*), the injurious effects of which are well known to most ranchers. Although comparatively new in the United States, it has been known in Europe for centuries. In ancient Greece, the Delphic oracle recommended its use as a cure for epilepsy.

Horn flies are a well-known pest of cattle throughout the length and breadth of the United States. The constant annoyance caused by these flies results in decreased weight and lessened milk production, and the loss from this source has been estimated at $10,000,000 annually. The horn fly was first recorded in this country near, Camden, N.J., in 1887. It is interesting to note that almost immediately preceding the appearance of this insect in New Jersey–in fact, the year before it was first observed–there was an extensive importation of Holstein cattle from Holland into that State. By the summer of 1889, the horn fly was recorded in Virginia, and it had established itself in Ohio by 1891. By 1892 it had spread northward into Canada and southwestward to eastern Texas. By 1895 it had covered practically all of the United States and Canada east of the Rocky Mountains, and 2 years later it was found in California and Oregon. Ten years from the time of its introduction, this pest had spread throughout North America and even to Hawaii.

In addition to the insects that attack our domestic animals, there is another group so closely associated with livestock that they are practically dependent on them for existence. In fact these insects rarely reproduce in noxious numbers in any substance other than the excreta of domestic animals. The most notorious is the housefly. The danger of contamination of dairy products by houseflies is now recognized in the milk laws of most States, which prohibit the sale of such products from premises where precautionary measures are not taken against the presence and breeding of houseflies. Compliance with these regulations involves huge expenditures of money and labour, but when the bacterial count in milk or cream is too high there is complete financial loss because the permit to sell is revoked.

Livestock Pests Not Yet Introduced into the United States

Though many livestock pests are quite cosmopolitan, many of the important ones known in other parts of the world have apparently not reached our shores. Among these might be mentioned the Golubatz fly (*Simulium columbaizense*), which is known to have caused the death of many thousands of wild and domesticated animals in Rumania in 1923. A botfly (*Hypoderma crossi*) seriously infests goats and occasionally attacks cattle in India. In the Union of Soviet Socialist Republics there is a fly (*Wohlfahrtia magnifica*) the larva of which injures the hoofs of animals. In the Philippines a foot maggot (*Booponus intonsus*) produces myiasis, a disease due to the presence of larvae; and in the Soviet Union a horse bot (*Rhinoestrus purpureus*), not known to occur in this country, causes considerable injury to horses. In parts of Africa, India, and the Philippines there is a screwworm (*Chrysomyia bezziana*) which, if introduced into this country, would greatly complicate our own screwworm problem, and already extensive damage is done to livestock here, by these pests. The well-known primary blowflies (*Calliphora stygia* and *C. augur*) of Australia, which breed in the soiled wool of sheep, might invade America if the right combination of circumstances was present. And last, but probably most serious of all, is the dreaded tsetse fly of Africa, which carries African sleeping sickness.

How Insect Pests Spread

The spread of insect pests of animals is definite and continuous. It is carried on in many different ways. For example, the tremendous swarms of adult buffalo gnats concentrating in the lower Mississippi Valley late in the spring, which have caused enormous losses of livestock, are hatched from eggs laid many hundreds of miles to the north and carried to the Mississippi lowlands on the crests of annual freshets.

It has been known that insect pests are carried great distances by the wind, but until collections were made by means of airplanes, the numbers and species that may be found at great heights were not fully comprehended. For example, a flea has been found 200 feet above the ground, mites and spiders at 1,000 feet and more, and flies and bees at an altitude of 14,000 feet–nearly 3 miles.

One of the most remarkable cases of insect spread by wind currents is that of a springtail, a primitive, wingless species, collected at an altitude of 3,000 feet. Although this insect was found over southern Louisiana, the species is known only in Cuba. Many of our most serious insect pests of animals are strong fliers in their own right and do not need the aid of wind currents for a change of scenery–witness the screwworm, which overwinters in southern Texas and flies northward on its own power approximately 35 miles a week, and the deer fly, which is one of our swiftest flying insects, although it does not travel far.

There are many other ways in which insect pests of animals may spread. It is not difficult to understand how easily ticks may be carried long distances in bales of hay or imported from outside the United States in guano; and the larvae and pupae of pests such as horn-flies, stableflies, and bots are commonly included in shipments of manure.

The common practice of shipping animals of all kinds long distances to agricultural fairs for exhibition and racing purposes gives their parasites easy and direct entry into new localities. The parasites of poultry are provided a safe and swift journey from their birthplace in eastern America when their hosts are sent to the west coast of the United States or Canada to take part in important egg-laying contests.

The movement of livestock to new ranges and new feed lots, and even to market, provides easy transportation for these insect pests from one section of the country to another and even across national boundaries. Modern passenger and express-carrying airplanes provide them with still another mode of travel.

Preventive Measures

Some of the measures that might aid in preventing the introduction of species or retarding those already established include quarantine and rigidly enforced inspection of both animals and their products, improved ranch management, and introduction of parasites and predators that prey only upon the injurious insects. In extreme instances it might become necessary to control certain parasites by temporary removal of their wild host.

It is generally known that many insect pests are controlled or their numbers greatly reduced by the introduction of their natural predators and parasites. The introduction of parasites of the eggs of horseflies into parts of Texas has been recorded as effectively reducing the numbers of these troublesome insects. Investigations have been made in Australia regarding this phase of control, apparently with some degree of success.

Wild animals sometimes harbour parasites that pass over to domestic species, causing injury and even death. In such cases it may be necessary to control the wild host or remove it entirely until control measures have been established for the injurious insect. A good example of this is the difficulty encountered in controlling the cattle tick in southern Florida. There it was found that the native white-tail deer served as a host for the southern cattle tick, and no matter how thoroughly the domestic animals were treated the wild reservoir continued to furnish sufficient numbers of ticks to prevent complete control. Unless quarantined, animals brought to this country for zoological gardens may easily bring their parasites along with them.

One of the important measures proposed by the Bureau of Entomology and Plant Quarantine for reducing screwworm losses is an improved form of ranch management which recommends timing of the birth of young and performing castration, docking, dehorning, and other surgical operations during the seasons when the screwworm fly is least abundant and least active.

Quarantines of sufficient duration should provide for thorough treatment of animals for such external parasites as lice, fleas, mites, ticks, and tick flies, and such internal parasites as bots, wound-infesting flies, and insect-borne protozoa, bacteria, and viruses. The time element is all-important, as bots, grubs, screwworms, and hoof maggots may spend more or less extended periods within their hosts and are not readily diagnosed from external examination. Certain forms of insects may emerge as adults even after their hosts have been in quarantine for 6 or 8 months. Proper precautions would allow these species to develop and emerge from their hosts while the animals are in quarantine, so that the pests can be destroyed.

Although quarantine regulations have caused many heated arguments and much dissatisfaction and are irksome and often difficult to apply, they are nevertheless exceedingly useful in preventing the spread of parasites as well as diseases.

A rigid and well-enforced inspection of animals entering interstate trade would prevent the transportation of screwworms by common carriers. Severe infestations of this insect have been started in the Central and Northern States by the shipment of infested animals from south Texas late in the spring. The local infestation then increases in size and importance until winter puts a stop to the depredations. An enforced inspection of animals in transit should be supplemented by a thorough cleaning and treatment of the common carrier and holding pens, as scab mites, ticks, fleas, and files could otherwise be carried to more distant points after their hosts have been unloaded.

At present the United States quarantine laws do not provide against the introduction of animal insect pests in the same thorough manner as against the importation of plant pests; they do, however, prohibit the importation of animals suffering from communicable diseases, some of which are transmitted by insects.

Chapter 10

REGULATORY ACTIVITIES IN ANIMAL-DISEASE CONTROL

A.W. Miller, S.O. Fladness, A.E. Wight, D.I. Skidmore, E.C. Joss, & H.E. Moskey[1]

[1] *A.W. Miller is Assistant Chief, Bureau of Animal Industry; S.O. Fladness is Chief, Field Inspection Division; A. E. Wight is Chief, Tuberculosis Eradication Division; D.I. Skidmore is Chief, Virus-Serum Control Division; and E.C. Joss is Chief, Meat Inspection Division; H.E. Moskey is Senior Veterinarian, Food and Drug Administration, Federal Security Agency.*

Certain Animal Diseases are so devastating when they gain a foothold that merciless war must be waged against them. No individual alone could protect his animals against these disease invasions; all must band together and take combined action through government. Here is the strategy of control, in which the real weapons are the findings of science.

Federal and State regulatory activities have a most important bearing on animal-disease control and eradication work. In fact such activities are often the foundation upon which programmes for the conduct of this work are built.

The first basic Federal legislation on this subject was the act approved May 29, 1884 (23 Stat. 31), which authorized the establishment of the Federal Bureau of Animal Industry. The purpose of this legislation was to prevent the exportation of diseased cattle and provide means for the suppression and wiping out of pleuro-pneumonia and other contagious diseases among domestic animals. This act contained authority for the promulgation of rules and regulations deemed necessary for the suppression of communicable diseases of livestock and also authorized the Department of Agriculture to establish quarantines.

At the time this legislation was enacted, the large export business in live cattle to Great Britain was endangered on account of the prevalence of contagious pleuro-pneumonia among cattle in the United States. The first great achievement in this country in completely eliminating a dangerous animal malady was the eradication of contagious pleuro-pneumonia, accomplished in 1892.

An amendment to the act of 1884, approved May 31, 1920 (41 Stat. 694, 699), contained a provision with respect to the interstate movement of cattle that had reacted to the tuberculin test. Another amendment, approved June 28, 1926 (44 Stat. 774), struck out provisions in the original act of 1884 under which it had been possible to ship cattle infested with cattle fever ticks across State lines. The effect of this amendment, which made it impossible to ship tick-infested cattle between States for immediate slaughter, was to provide a much-needed stimulus to tick-eradication work, especially in some areas where it had been lagging.

The act of February 2, 1903 (32 Stat. 791), was passed to enable the Department more effectually to suppress and prevent contagious and infectious diseases of livestock. The act of March 3, 1905 (33 Stat. 1264), broadened the authority of the Secretary of Agriculture to establish and maintain quarantine districts and to permit and regulate the movement of cattle and other livestock therefrom.

The acts of August 30, 1890, and February 2, 1903, as well as provisions in various appropriation acts, gave the Secretary of Agriculture additional authority to prescribe regulations for the inspection (Fig. 1) and quarantine of livestock offered for importation and for control and supervision over such imported products as hay, straw, etc., which are possible conveyers of infection. These regulations are modified from time to time as new knowledge is developed regarding conditions under which the various infections will survive for long periods and the manner in which they are disseminated.

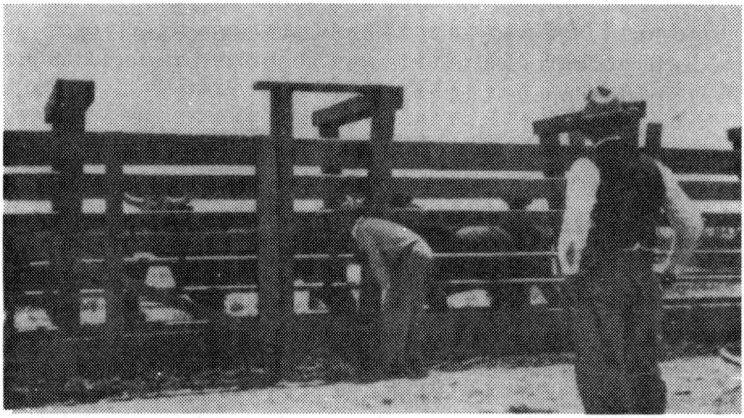

Fig. 1: Inspection of import cattle from.Mexico. Inspection is made principally to see whether any cattle ticks are present. The high, strong chute makes possible close inspection of the animals, many of which are semiwild and unaccustomed to being handled.

In safeguarding livestock producers in the United States from losses due to animal diseases it is essential that every possible effort be made to prevent the introduction of foreign animal maladies, to stamp out promptly any infection that may gain a foothold, and to employ comprehensive and adequate measures in combating diseases that have been long establishment in this country.

If the contagion of any disease normally nonexistent in this country is introduced and threatens the livestock industry, the Secretary has authority to cooperate with the States concerned in drastic eradication measures, including the purchase and destruction of diseased or exposed animals and contaminated materials.

Among the more important regulatory features that have been of material assistance in the work of combating for animal diseases are Federal and State quarantines; campaigns for disease control and eradication; the keeping of records to disclose the extent and distribution of various maladies; and public-stock-yards inspection, including testing livestock before interstate shipment, cleaning and disinfecting premises and vehicles, immunization of swine against hog cholera, dipping of cattle and sheep for scabies, and the enforcement of the so-called 28-hour law. Supervision over the production of biological products and control of drug remedies are also important phases of the work.

Federal and State Quarantines

Federal and State quarantines are of very great value in campaigns for the control and eradication of animal diseases. These measures are usually put into effect through the issuance of rules and regulations based on legislation which in many instances is general but which confers on the enforcing officer ample authority to prescribe definite and detailed specifications for the work.

In combating most infectious diseases of livestock the stoppage of the movement of diseased and exposed animals is essential. This can seldom be accomplished without some kind of quarantine. The principal object for the establishment of any quarantine is to confine the infection to the smallest possible area and to hold it there until it can be stamped out through the use of appropriate eradication measures. The problem of protecting our herds and flocks has been greatly simplified by the fact that several of the most serious communicable diseases of animals have not gained a permanent foothold in this country.

Sometimes it is possible to prevent a highly infectious disease from gaining a foothold by the strict enforcement of a local quarantine. This is well demonstrated by the practice of holding animals offered for importation into the United States in quarantine at ports of entry for a period of observation. This practice in a number of instance has prevented the introduction of foreign animal maladies into this country, the most noteworthy case having been the detection of surra in a consignment of Brahman cattle on arrival in the United States. The detection of the disease in this instance and the slaughter of the affected animals made it possible to maintain the record of never having had an outbreak of surra in the herds of this country.

Rinderpest has never gained entrance into the United States. Foot-and-mouth disease has been brought in six times since the Bureau of Animal Industry was organized, but in each instance complete eradication has been successfully accomplished. The United States has remained free from mal de caderas of horses and several other destructive maladies which, along with surra, are caused by a class of organisms known as trypanosomes.

When an outbreak of foot-and-mouth disease occurs it is the practice of both the Federal and the State officials concerned to impose drastic quarantine measures. These not only prohibit all movement from infected premises but in addition prohibit or greatly restrict the movement within the quarantined area of livestock and materials considered likely to serve as means for the spread of the disease. Usually the borders of a quarantine established on account of foot-and-mouth disease are identical in the quarantine orders issued by the Federal and the State authorities. In some instances the State may, as a precautionary measure, establish a modified quarantine area around the infected area from which a limited movement of animals and farm products is permitted under close supervision of the State sanitary officials.

When the disease to be combated is not especially virulent and has not become widespread, it is possible to handle outbreaks by the application of State quarantines without the imposition of a Federal quarantine. When the disease has become widespread and well established, however, local quarantines are not adequate, especially when it is necessary to regulate the movement of livestock and vehicles used in their transportation from an entire State or a number of States. In such instances a Federal quarantine is imposed, and the interested States cooperate by putting State quarantines in effect, as was done in the campaigns to eradicate sheep and cattle scabies, southern or splenetic fever tick, and foot-and-mouth disease.

To be effective and to have the support of interested agencies, especially of livestock producers, quarantine measures must vary greatly and be appropriate for the particular disease that is being combated. They may range from a complete prohibition against the movement of all animals, produce, and vehicles, and even restrictions on human beings, as in the case of an outbreak of foot-and-mouth disease, to mere physical examination and movement under proper certification or official permit, as in the case of sheep and cattle scab; in which the animals are subjected to certain prescribed treatments that have been found to be effective.

While the campaign for the eradication of tuberculosis was at its height, regulations were issued by cities, counties, and some States prohibiting the sale of any butter or other dairy products not produced from cream or milk obtained from cattle from non-infected dairy herds in the modified tuberculosis-free area. Although these were not technically quarantine measures, the results very noticeably hastened the work of eradicating bovine tuberculosis.

The cooperation of livestock producers in the enforcement of quarantine measures, both State and Federal, usually has been excellent, although in a few instances it has been necessary to employ armed guards in order to maintain an effective quarantine.

Since quarantine measures interfere in varying degrees with the operations of livestock producers, they should be imposed only when other means would be ineffective and lifted as promptly as conditions warrant. It would be impossible, however, to control and eradicate some of the contagious diseases in this country without the authority, both Federal and State, to impose quarantines.

Campaigns for Disease Control and Eradication

A long-term programme of eradication, undertaken county by county and State by State with active cooperation between Federal and State livestock sanitary organizations, livestock producers, and others, is commonly called a campaign.

Although some of the most dangerous diseases have been successfully excluded, a number of others unfortunately had become widely disseminated and were serious deterrents to the livestock industry before there were means for dealing with them effectively. These diseases, which included hog cholera, scabies (mange), splenetic or tick fever, dourine of horses, and bovine tuberculosis, naturally engaged the attention of the Bureau of Animal Industry very soon after its organization. Through careful study and research important gaps in the knowledge of the causative agents and their characteristics and mode of transmission were gradually filled in and the foundation was thus laid for the next step, which was to devise means for combating the diseases mentioned. In this step, too, the investigators achieved notable results. Methods were developed which rendered possible the complete elimination of all the diseases except hog cholera.

The act of Congress approved May 29, 1884, which created the Bureau of Animal Industry, also provided authority for the Secretary of Agriculture to cooperate with the various States in the eradication of diseases and prescribed conditions under which such cooperation may be extended. That law has been supplemented from time to time by other statutes, including provisions in annual-appropriation acts, in regard to special problems that have arisen in dealing with particular diseases. Accordingly, as fast as practicable and effective methods have been devised and the specified conditions fulfilled in the different States concerned, cooperative eradication projects have been organized and systematic work done on as large a scale as available funds and personnel have made possible from year to year. The first of these extensive cooperative programmes to be, undertaken was the eradication of scabies of cattle and sheep in the great range areas of the West. This was begun in 1905. The following year witnessed the inauguration of the campaign to eradicate the ticks which transmit splenetic or tick fever, then prevalent in all the Southern States. Intensive efforts to eliminate dourine date from 1912, and the eradication of bovine tuberculosis, the most extensive and costly of all the programmes to date, got under way in 1911. All these campaigns are now nearing completion.

Objectives in Campaigns Combating Animal Diseases

While complete eradication is the final objective in all of these campaigns, two quite different principles are involved which call for correspondingly different methods and procedures. Scabies and tick fever, for instance, are caused or transmitted by external parasites, and eradication must be accomplished by treatment of the affected animals for the destruction of the parasites. On the other hand, the presence or absence of dourine and tuberculosis is determined by diagnostic tests, and animals found to be infected are appraised and slaughtered. Owners of destroyed animals are indemnified by the Department and the cooperating State or local government, within certain limits fixed by the governing laws and regulations.

The manner in which hog cholera is dealt with in the United States represents another form of cooperative effort. The existence of that disease was general throughout the country, and widespread epizootics (equivalent to epidemics in the case of human disease) more or less regularly caused enormous losses. Early in the present century scientists of the Bureau of Animal Industry determined the cause of hog cholera and devised a practical and reliable method of rendering swine immune to the disease. Cooperative projects were set up in a majority of the States to demonstrate the application of the method and promote its general use, along with indicated sanitary measures. This project, inaugurated in 1913, aimed at control and prevention rather than eradication.

The efforts toward the control and eradication of communicable animal diseases within the different States are primarily the function of the respective State authorities. The direct authority of the Federal Government extends only to control over the interstate movement of livestock from districts where any such disease is known to prevail. Authority to enforce local quarantines and to compel the destruction or the treatment of infected or exposed animals rests entirely with the States. Consequently, the work of these Federal and State cooperative projects is one chiefly under State laws and regulations. Cooperative work as contemplated by section 3 of the act of May 29, 1884, is not undertaken in any State unless or until there are State laws and regulations which make it possible to apply established methods effectively and to protect the results achieved and unless State authorities undertake to proceed in harmony with the general policies and practices agreed upon by Federal and State livestock sanitary authorities.

It will be apparent from the foregoing that in formulating plans for dealing with communicable diseases of livestock the objective to be sought is a primary consideration.

In the case of tick fever and scabies the course to be followed is very clear. Methods of eradication have been developed which, if properly carried out, are completely effective. In the case of some diseases, however, no means of accomplishing complete eradication have been found. In others, while eradication might be possible it would be quite impracticable to attempt it, either because the cost would be prohibitive or because effective and economical methods of control are available. In still others, no such methods of control have been developed, and eradication is possible and feasible if prompt and thorough action is taken before the disease has gained too strong a foothold.

Anthrax and blackleg are examples of diseases that are not susceptible of eradication but losses from which can be largely prevented through the prophylactic treatment of susceptible animals in infected areas, along with collateral sanitary measures. An example of a disease which can be eradicated but which it is most often more feasible to control is hog cholera. In Canada, where the disease rarely appears, the occasional outbreaks that do occur are eradicated by the prompt slaughter of all swine in affected herds, followed by disinfection of the premises. In the United States, on the other hand, in view of the fact that hog cholera exists in all regions and the further fact that swine can be effectively protected against it, a policy of prevention and control was indicated and is being followed.

Foot-and-mouth disease and hog cholera, as they are dealt with in this country, furnish the most striking illustrations of the application of the policies of eradication and control. Both diseases are caused by viruses, those minute organisms that are invisible under the strongest microscope, pass through the finest filters, and can be cultivated only in living tissues-characteristics which render diseases caused by them unusually difficult to deal with. Both are eradicable if extreme measures are taken before the virus has become too widely disseminated. In other respects they are quite dissimilar. The hog cholera virus causes disease only in swine, whereas all ruminants as well as swine are susceptible to foot-and-mouth disease. Losses from hog cholera can be reduced to the varnishing point through the application of control measures of proved efficiency. On, the other hand, experience in European countries where foot-and-mouth disease is always present has demonstrated that when the virus is widespread effective control of the disease is not possible. Consequently, when an outbreak of foot-and-mouth disease occurs in the United States there is no choice but to proceed with eradication, no matter how drastic the measures that must be taken.

The practical impossibility of controlling foot-and-mouth disease where it exists enzootically–that is, where there are always a few cases in the animal population-may be ascribed to a combination of factors. Probably first among these is the fact that it is the most infectious disease of animals known and spreads with extreme rapidity. Another factor is the existence of several types of the virus and the fact that immunity resulting from infection by one type does not protect animals exposed to other types. Still another factor is the failure thus far to develop an immunizing product at once effective against all types of the virus and practicable for use on a large scale, without which no adequate control over the disease when it exists extensively can be hoped for. This situation pointedly illustrates the need, in the United States, for adhering to the policy of complete eradication of any outbreaks that may occur.

Public-Stockyards Inspection

The closing decade of the nineteenth century and the first of the twentieth witnessed a tremendous growth of public markets in the United States and the development of a considerable number of additional stockyards for the receipt of livestock from all parts of the country. Some of these were for disposition for immediate slaughter; others were for reshipment after sale to widely scattered country points for feeding, stocking, or breeding purposes. Realizing that the intermingling of the tremendous numbers of animals involved might cause these market places to become centers of infection from which serious animal maladies would be spread to ranches and farms throughout the country, the Department set up an inspection service which has proved to be an important factor in the campaign to control and eradicate animal diseases. This service is separate and distinct from ante mortem inspection at slaughtering establishments where Federal meat inspection is maintained. Although often adjacent to meat-packing establishments, public stock-yards are separately managed.

Livestock-inspection service is maintained at 48 stockyards in 46 cities. Veterinarians who, through years of experience, have become skilled in the detection of animals affected with disease or other abnormal conditions are constantly on duty examining the animals that pass through these stockyards each day. These veterinarians are assisted by laymen skilled in such work as the inspection of livestock, supervising the dipping of cattle and sheep for scabies, and cleaning and disinfecting premises, cars, and trucks used in the handling of diseased animals.

So far as possible all livestock that arrive at these market centers during daylight hours are inspected at the time of unloading, while animals that are unloaded and yarded during the night are inspected early in the morning before the trading commences.

Among the principal diseases for which inspections are made are anthrax, scabies of cattle and sheep, tick or splenetic fever, hog cholera, hemorrhagic septicemia (shipping fever), and erysipelas of swine. If signs of these or any other communicable disease are detected, all infected and exposed animals are promptly segregated and treated or otherwise handled in accordance with Department regulations. The inspectors are constantly on the watch for animals showing any symptoms suspicious of foot-and-mouth disease.

The livestock sanitary official of the State in which a diseased shipment originates is notified, as well as the Department field office in that territory. In this way centers of infection are located, and the spread of the disease to other herds and premises is frequently prevented by the prompt application of appropriate sanitary control measures. Instances are not uncommon in which the detection of disease in a shipment at a public stockyard is the owner's first inkling of the existence of infection on his premises.

Not only are incoming shipments of livestock inspected, but a reinspection is made of outgoing shipments, both to detect disease and also to determine whether there has been compliance with certain requirements, such as the tests for tuberculosis and Bang's disease, dipping for scabies, and immunization against hog cholera.

The very large scale on which this livestock-inspection service is conducted is indicated by the fact that each year there pass through these public markets for slaughter or other purposes between 60 and 70 million head of livestock, the figures for the fiscal year 1940 being 18,135,667 cattle, 21,832,485 sheep, and 29,540,954 swine. As an indication of the importance of this service, the detection at one market during the calendar year 1940 of more than 160 consignments of sheep affected with scabies may be cited.

Testing Livestock Before Interstate Shipment

Interstate shipments of livestock for immediate slaughter may be made to public stockyards under regulations that are less restrictive than if the animals are to be forwarded direct from some country point in one State to a country point in another State for feeding, stocking, or breeding purposes. If, however, it is found after arrival that some of the animals would sell to better advantage for the latter purposes than for slaughter, they then must meet the same test requirements that would have been applicable if they had been shipped direct for such purposes.

Department employees at public stockyards supervise the application of the tests for tuberculosis and Bang's disease and see that those animals which do not pass a satisfactory test are removed from the consignments to which they belong and are slaughtered or otherwise properly disposed of, as may be prescribed in existing regulations. The bulk of all the cattle that react to the tests for tuberculosis and Bang's disease in the present cooperative Federal and State campaign are sent to these public markets for slaughter. The employees at the markets exercise the utmost vigilance to see that the identity of these reactors, estimated at 180,000 in 1940, is maintained during their passage through the yards and that they are sold and finally disposed of for immediate slaughter.

Cleaning and Disinfection

Whenever disease is found in a shipment of livestock to these public markets, immediate steps are taken to see that the pens occupied by the animals at the market, the car or other vehicle in which they have been transported (Fig. 2), and the yards through which they have been handled at the point of origin–and en route if they have been unloaded for feed, water, and rest-are properly cleaned and disinfected.

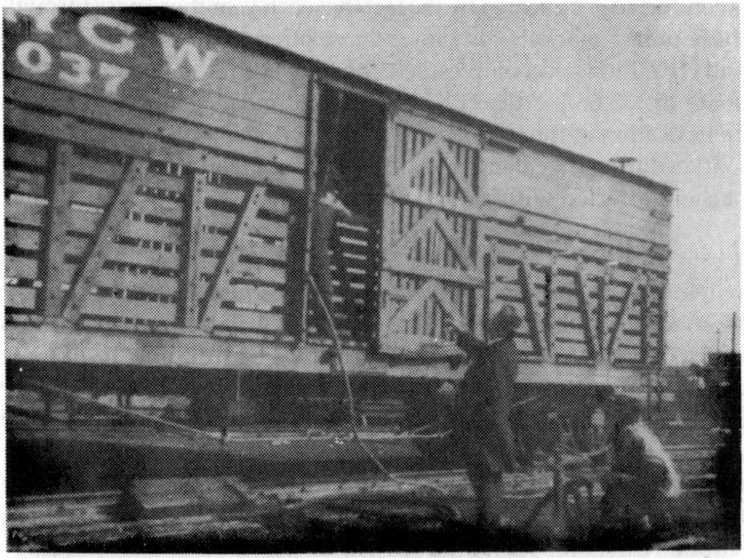

Fig. 2: A Government veterinarian supervising the cleaning and disinfection of a stock car that had carried tuberculous cattle. The airtight container at the right contains the disinfecting solution and is provided with a pressure gage and valve to admit compressed air, brought to the spot by underground pipes. The air pressure, controlled by a valve, forces the disinfectant through the hose, which is fitted with a nozzle for spraying the inside of the car.

Immunization and Dipping

Another activity over which the Department exercises supervision at public stockyards is the immunization of swine against hog cholera. Included in receipts at many of the large markets, especially at certain times of the year, are a considerable number of pigs which are not in first-class slaughter condition. Under the regulations in effect it is possible to sort out such animals from the consignments in which they are received and sell them for shipment to country points for further feeding, provided they are properly treated against hog cholera.

Such swine may be moved interstate from public stockyards for any purpose only to States the laws, rules, and regulations of which provide for the segregation and quarantine of imported hogs for a period of not less than 3 weeks. In order to be eligible for such shipment certain inspection and certification requirements must be met. The swine must be inspected by a Bureau inspector at the yards. If they are found free from symptoms of cholera or other contagious, infectious, or communicable diseases and in a thrifty condition, they must be treated by a competent veterinarian under Bureau supervision, provided that the temperature of each animal is taken before treatment and that only those with a temperature of less than 104° F. shall be permitted interstate movement. If the Bureau inspector finds any hogs affected with cholera, the entire lot to which they belong must be treated by a competent veterinarian under Bureau supervision in a portion of the yards set aside for that purpose. At the expiration of not less than 30 days, if no signs of disease are observed on examination of the hogs, they may be released for shipment. All immunized swine must be disinfected by dipping in or spraying with a permitted solution, must be accompanied by a certificate issued by a Bureau inspector, and must be transported in cleaned and disinfected cars or other vehicles.

These swine in many instances originate in localities where feed supplies are short, often because of drought conditions, and they are usually sold at stockyards to purchasers who in most instances are located in sections which at the time have surplus feed. The immunization of these animals, therefore, is of value not only to the producer, who is afforded an outlet for his unfinished animals, but also to the purchaser, who needs additional animals to consume the feed he has available.

Consignments of sheep and cattle received at public stockyards in which scabies infection is found or which have been exposed to the disease, if not sold for immediate slaughter, are dipped in accordance with applicable regulations under Department supervision. Included in the receipts of sheep at these stockyards are many animals not in a fit condition for slaughter. These are sorted out of their consignments and sold for feeding or breeding purposes. Many of them are dipped as a precautionary measure to comply with the requirements of the States to which they are destined or at the request of the purchasers, even though there is no actual knowledge that they have been exposed to scabies. This dipping also is conducted under Department supervision.

Meat Inspection as an Aid in Animal-Disease-Control Activities

An important service of the Bureau of Animal Industry is the administration of the Federal meat-inspection laws. The purpose of the inspection is to protect consumers of meat and meat food products, so far as the Federal Government has legislated, against bad meats and against insanitary conditions and deceptive and fraudulent practices during the preparation of meat products for the channels of commerce.

Some 70,000,000 or more cattle, sheep, swine, and goats are submitted each year to this inspection. These animals, if lined up closely in single file, would encircle the world at the Equator more than 2½ times; yet, as they daily flow into federally inspected establishments each animal is inspected twice before its transformation into meat is completed.

Inspection procedure is as follows:

First, the animals are scrutinized and if necessary examined more closely in the pens of the establishment in order that those that are sick or for some other reason are unfit for human food purposes may be sorted out and destroyed or otherwise properly disposed of. Although a very large percentage of these animals have passed through public stockyards and have been inspected there, these establishments are not a part of the yards and this ante mortem inspection is distinct from the public-stockyards inspection.

Second, as the animals passed on the ante mortem inspection are slaughtered and dressed in the establishment, each carcass with its parts, including the internal organs, is inspected for signs of disease or other conditions which render the meat unsafe or objectionable as food.

Third, hams, bacon, lard, sausage, canned meats, and other food products of the meat and organs are marked "U.S. Inspected and Passed" after post mortem inspection.

The ante mortem and post mortem inspections form the main stem of the Federal system of inspection, and to conduct this part of the service more than 800 veterinarians are regularly employed, along with a somewhat smaller number of trained lay inspectors as assistants.

Through a system of daily reports by the veterinarians who make the ante mortem and post mortem inspections, a record is available of the affected animals and carcasses examined and disposed of. These records have value other than as mere statistics. For example, when a veterinarian engaged in meat inspection finds an animal or a shipment of animals affected with a communicable disease of importance to livestock sanitary officials and when he can ascertain the origin of the diseased animal or animals, he reports the circumstances directly to the State or Federal sanitary officials having jurisdiction in the region from which the infected livestock came. By means of eartags, earmarks, brands, tattoo marks, or even descriptions of animals, the center of infection is often located, with quick and beneficial results to the livestock owners in the vicinity. The veterinary meat-inspection records are also useful to research scientists and others in ascertaining the location and spread of animal diseases in various regions of the country.

The Act to Prevent Cruelty to Animals in Transit

The act to prevent cruelty to animals in transit–the so-called 28-hour law–although not designed primarily for the control of animal diseases, does have such a direct influence on the health of livestock that it merits a discussion in this article. This measure has general application throughout the United States, but most of the work in connection with its enforcement is performed at public stockyards.

Department employees at such yards examine waybills, interview shippers, and in other ways endeavour to discover alleged violations of this law. Any cases that appear suspicious are thoroughly investigated, and if sufficient evidence to warrant prosecution is found, the violation is reported to the Department, which sends it through the Office of its solicitor to the Department of Justice for prosecution.

This act prohibits railroads or other common carriers from confining cattle, sheep, swine, or other animals shipped across State lines for longer than 28 hours without unloading into properly equipped pens (Fig. 3) for feed, water, and rest for a period of 5 hours, unless prevented by storm or other accidental or unavoidable causes which could not be anticipated or avoided by the exercise of due diligence and foresight. The law contains a provision that on written request of the shipper the time of confinement may be extended to 36 hours. The provisions of this law, which was enacted in 1906 before motor transportation had come into general use, have been held not to apply to animals moved interstate in trucks. An

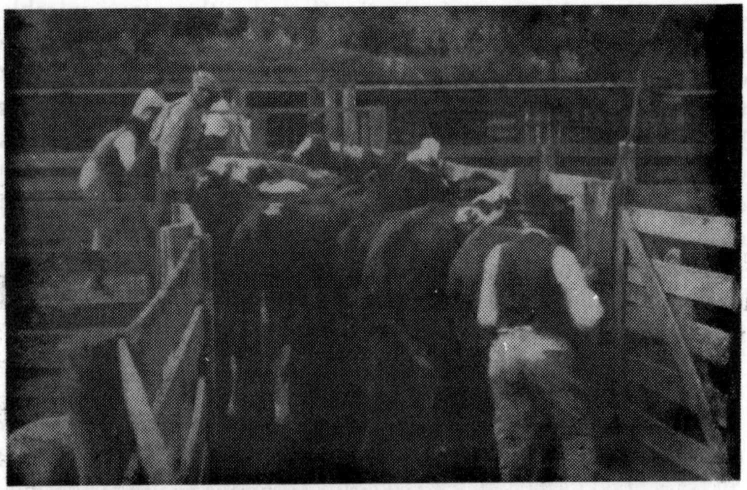

Fig. 3. Cattle on their way to market leaving railway rest pens to be reloaded in cars. Before the enactment of the 28-hour law, livestock were often confined in cars for long periods without water, feed, or rest. Such conditions sapped the vitality of the animals, many of them arriving at their destination exhausted or sick, or even crippled. Deaths in transit were also much more frequent than under present improved conditions.

effort is being made to have the law amended to cover this new development in livestock transportation.

For a number of years following the enactment of this measure a great deal of difficulty was experienced in enforcing it. Opposition was encountered from both the railroads and the shippers of livestock. However, as it was gradually realized that livestock would reach market in better condition if the law were observed, violations dropped off. Today the Department has the hearty cooperation of practically all the railroads in the United States, and violations are relatively few.

Enforcement of the act has resulted in the provision by railroads of more adequate facilities at feed, water, and rest stations and the expediting of the movement of livestock to avoid penalties for infractions of the law. On a number of occasions efforts have been made to amend the law so that the time of confinement could be extended to 40 hours. In the opinion of the Department such a provision would be an unwise one and detrimental to the interests of the shipper, especially as the vitality of animals that are deprived of feed, water, and rest for long periods is lowered and they thus become more likely to develop diseases such as hemorrhagic septicemia.

Regulation of Biological Products

The virus-serum-toxin law of March 1913 authorizes the Secretary of Agriculture to make and promulgate such rules and regulations as may be necessary to prevent the preparation, sale, barter, exchange, or interstate shipment of worthless, contaminated, dangerous, or harmful viruses, serums, toxins, or analogous products for use in the treatment of domestic animals. Under this authority Bureau of Animal Industry Order 276 and its amendments have been issued. The main purpose of these regulations is to insure that there will be available for the treatment of livestock such serums, vaccines, diagnostic agents, and like biological products as will assist in effectively preventing controlling, or eradicating diseases that threaten the health of the farmer's domestic animals and indirectly his livelihood.

Biological products that are contaminated or not properly prepared or used may fail to prevent or control an outbreak of disease or may even be the means of spreading disease, endangering not only the animals on the farm on which they are used but perhaps other herds in the community. Biological products produced under licenses issued by the Secretary and in accordance with his regulations carry reasonable assurance that if they are properly applied and their use is restricted as indicated by the trade label they will be effective as an aid in preventing the specific disease named on the label and will not be harmful to the farmer's animals on which they are used or endanger those of other owners.

During the last year a sufficient quantity of anti-hog-cholera serum was produced by licensed establishments under Department regulations to treat more than 33,000,000 shoats. It is not difficult to imagine what would have happened had any considerable part of this serum been worthless or impotent or contaminated with the causative agent of a dangerous communicable disease of animals. Biological products that do not meet requirements are with held from the market and destroyed under the supervision of Bureau inspectors.

From time to time the regulations have been amended or supplemented with orders designed to improve the quality of biological products marketed by licensed establishments. Whenever new tests are developed, licensed producers are required to subject their products to these tests and to market none that are found unsatisfactory. Likewise, when new production procedures are developed, they are applied to products to improve their quality.

A considerable part of the supervision exercised over establishments producing biological products under license involves the proper labeling of each product. The purpose of the regulations relating to labeling is to prevent misbranding by insuring as far as possible that the products are properly identified by name and descriptive matter, that adequate directions are given for the proper use of each product, and that no statement, design, or device that may deceive the purchaser or that is false and misleading in any particular is used.

Drug Remedies and Their Control

Naturally desiring healthy livestock but lacking knowledge of diseases and the limitations of drugs in preventing and treating diseases, many farmers have been led to spend much money for remedies of no value whatever. Though there are no exact figures on the subject, it has been estimated that farmers spend many millions of dollars each year on livestock and poultry remedies, in spite of the fact that the value of drug medication in the prevention and treatment of infectious diseases caused by bacterial agents and filterable viruses is extremely limited. In addition to involving a monetary loss, the use of worthless remedies gives farmers a false sense of security.

Scientists all over the world have spent much time seeking to discover chemicals or drugs that when administered internally would destroy the causative agents of infectious or communicable diseases of livestock without being topic to the tissues or organs of the body. Up to the present time veterinary authorities know of no chemical or drugs that have been scientifically established as being effective in the prevention or treatment of any of the specific diseases of animals caused by bacteria or filterable viruses. Valuable discoveries have been made by scientists in the treatment of certain specific bacterial infections in man with the sulfanilamide compounds, but unfortunately, this group of drugs has not fulfilled the expectation of veterinarians in the treatment of bacterial diseases of livestock, including poultry.

This is not to say that all drugs are worthless in the treatment of animals. Many have physiological or therapeutic effects that have been more or less well established scientifically. These drugs are not used or prescribed with the idea that they will remove or destroy the bacterial or virus infection or prevent the disease from spreading to other animals. They are useful for their known effects on the tissues or organs of the body, and their use may be highly desirable in the treatment of sick animals. For example, powdered nux vomica and gentian are the basic drugs in many livestock tonics. A combination of drugs of this character when prescribed in therapeutically significant amounts is scientifically recognized to have a stimulating effect on appetite and tone, but it will not be effective in removing the cause of any disease condition. Likewise the drug digitalis is valuable for its specific action on the heart, but its use will not correct any abnormal condition of the heart.

The combination of iron and copper is frequently prescribed for its effect in increasing the hemoglobin content of the blood. This treatment is especially useful in cases of anemia associated with a deficiency of iron and copper in the diet, but it is not effective in the removal of other causes of anemia. Supplementing the ration with certain minerals and vitamins in which the feed is known to be deficient has been recognized by scientists to be effective in correcting abnormal conditions associated with particular mineral or vitamin deficiencies. A good example of the real value of certain minerals is the treatment of the disease of cattle known as milk fever, which is associated with a calcium deficiency. This condition responds almost immediately to injections of sterile calcium compounds into the veins or under the skin. On the other hand, unscrupulous manufacturers of mineral mixtures and vitamin preparations have attempted, by advertising, to create the unwarranted and misleading impression that products of this nature are of value in the control of infectious diseases and worm infestation.

In recent years internal parasites of animals have received considerable attention from veterinary investigators in this country as well as elsewhere. A number of specific drug treatments have been discovered, particularly by the United States Bureau of Animal Industry. A notable example is the new drug phenothiazine. No known drug or combination of drugs, however, will remove all species of worms from all species of animals. As a rule, these drugs are specific in their effects in each species of animal for each species of worm.

Laymen commonly believe that because a drug is effective for certain types of worms in one animal it will be equally effective for similar types of worms in other animals. This is a mistaken idea. The drug arecoline hydrobromide, for example, is effective in the removal of the common species of tapeworms from dogs, but it has not been found to be effective in the removal of the common species of tapeworms infesting chickens. Another example is the drug nicotine, or powdered tobacco containing nicotine, which has proved to be effective for the removal of large roundworms from poultry but has not been found to be of any value in removing large roundworms from hogs, dogs, or horses.

Livestock and poultry raisers have been more or less familiar with the activities of the Food and Drug Administration in the enforcement of the Food and Drugs Act of 1906. In the past 15 years, the Administration has issued approximately 500 Notices of Judgment concerning misbranded livestock remedies on which seizure and prosecution cases were terminated by the Federal courts.

During this time, thousands of samples have been collected and analyzed. Many of these were simple inexpensive drugs disguised in different ways. Others contained many drugs in minute amounts. One preparation consisted of cornstarch with just enough potassium permanganate to make a pink solution in water. It was represented as a treatment for Bang's disease and sold for $5 to $12 a package.

The article had no value whatever in the treatment of any disease. This case, like many similar cases, was referred by the Food and Drug Administration to the Department of Justice for criminal prosecution. While in most of the Food and Drug cases the defendant enters a plea of guilty, the case referred to was contested by the defendant and tried before a jury, which found him guilty of misbranding his product.

Such activities of the Food and Drug Administration have resulted in the disappearance from interstate channels of misbranded drug remedies represented to be effective for the prevention and treatment of Bang's disease, mastitis or garget, sterility or breeding troubles, hog cholera, swine fever, hog influenza, "necro" (necrotic enteritis), mixed infections, influenza of horses, horse distemper, strangles, sleeping sickness of horses, fowl cholera, chickenpox, coccidiosis, roup, bronchitis, fowl paralysis, pullorum disease, blackhead of turkeys, distemper, running fits, and blacktongue of dogs, and the prevention of intestinal worms.

Recent Food and Drug Legislation

On June 25, 1938, Congress enacted the new Federal Food, Drug, and Cosmetic Act designed to replace the act of 1906 and to provide for more effective control. The Food and Drug Administration, which is charged with the enforcement of this act, was transferred on June 30, 1940, from the Department of Agriculture to the Federal Security Agency.

Farmers should know that the Federal Food, Drug, and Cosmetic Act gives the Food and Drug Administration no authority to regulate veterinary remedies sold within the State in which they are manufactured and no control over advertising matter distributed separately from the product. The recently enacted Wheeler-Lea Act, which is enforced by the Federal Trade Commission, does give that Commission authority to regulate advertising of foods, drugs, and cosmetics for man or animals; and the Post Office Department has authority to prevent fraudulent use of the mails in the sale of livestock and poultry remedies.

The Food, Drug, and Cosmetic Act of 1938 contains several new provisions which should be of interest to the purchasing public.

The term "device" under the new act is defined to mean "instruments, apparatus, and contrivances, including their components, parts, and accessories, intended (1) for use in the diagnosis, cure, mitigation, treatment, or prevention of disease in man or other animals; (2) to affect the structure or any function of the body of man or other animals."

For example, owners of dogs have been led to believe that certain chemically treated, copper-lined collars when worn by dogs win prevent or cure mange. For cattle wooden plugs or metal tubes intended to be inserted into the wombs of cows have been represented as a means of correcting breeding troubles. Such devices are not only of no value but may even be injurious.

Before any new drug can legitimately be shipped in interstate commerce, the manufacturer is required under the act to file an application with the Administrator of the Federal Security Agency, giving a full report of investigations that have been made to show whether or not the drug is safe for use. Interstate shipments of drugs dangerous to the health of livestock and poultry when used in the dosage or with the frequency or duration prescribed, recommended, or suggested in the labeling thereof are prohibited. The act requires the labeling of drugs and devices to bear warnings against probable misuse which may be dangerous to health; it also requires special precautionary labeling for drugs that are liable to deterioration. The act also prohibits interstate traffic in drugs that have been prepared or handled under insanitary conditions whereby they may have been contaminated with filth or that may have rendered the contents injurious to health. Drug remedies when shipped in interstate commerce must bear in a conspicuous manner on the main or principal display panel of the label the common or usual name of each active ingredient, including quantities or proportions of certain specified drugs. The label also must bear an accurate statement of the quantity of the contents in terms of weight, measure, or numerical count and the name and address of the manufacturer, packer, or distributor. By one of the most important provisions of the act a drug is deemed misbranded if its labeling is false or misleading in any particular. Since livestock and poultry feeds also are subject to the Federal Food, Drug, and Cosmetic Act the Food and Drug Administration actively cooperates with the State feed officials in the removal of adulterated or misbranded feeds from the channels of interstate commerce.

Drugs represented as useful for the treatment and control of insects infesting animals, as well as disinfectants for contaminated premises or objects, are subject to the Federal Insecticide Act of 1910. These types of products when shipped in interstate commerce are under constant surveillance to see that they will do all that is claimed for them in the labeling material. Like the Food, Drug, and Cosmetic Act, the Insecticide Act gives the Federal Government no authority to regulate such products when sold within the State in which they are manufactured or over advertising material distributed separately from the product. The Insecticide Act was formerly enforced by the Food and Drug Administration, but since June 30, 1940, it has been enforced by the Agricultural Marketing Service of the Department of Agriculture.

Chapter 11

FIGHTING DISEASE WITH KNOWLEDGE

D.S. Burch[1]

[1] *D.S. Burch is Agricultural Editor and Assistant to the Chief of the Bureau of Animal Industry, in charge of publications and related information work.*

"The most successful livestock owners appear to have prospered in large measure because they have built up effective barriers against disease, utilized veterinary services, and otherwise sought to reduce losses from the inroads of diseases and pests." Knowledge, the author holds, is the first step toward this kind of success, and supplying knowledge is one of the basic functions of public agencies concerned with disease control.

Factual information concerning animal diseases is of paramount value in dealing with them intelligently and effectively. Veterinary science has already provided such information concerning most animal maladies and is steadily adding to the reservoirs of useful scientific knowledge. Because science is altruistic, it has made its findings available to all people throughout the world, largely in the form of published literature.

Veterinary Education and Service

To provide for the application of scientific knowledge through professional services, veterinary colleges have utilized published information in training students to engage in private practice or to serve the public in inspection work, research, or other technical capacities. In the school year 1941-42, 10 colleges in the United States and 2 in Canada offered degrees in veterinary medicine on completion, of a 4-year course. In recent years enrollment in these 12 colleges has ranged from about 2,100 to 2,400 students, and their graduates have numbered 400 to 500 annually. All the other countries in the world have a total of 13 veterinary colleges and schools. Most veterinarians in the United States are graduates of the North American institutions. In all States the practice of veterinary medicine is regulated by laws with which veterinarians must comply before they may legally pursue their profession. In most States applicants must pass examinations or licensing tests in order to engage in veterinary practice.

According to census data and supplemental estimates, the United States has approximately 12,000 veterinarians, of whom about two-thirds are in private practice. The remainder are engaged in Federal, State, county, and municipal inspection activities or research, teaching, or commercial work. In relation to the number of veterinarians it is noteworthy that there are approximately 5 million livestock producers in the United States and that the number of cattle, horses, swine, sheep, and goats is normally about 200 million. On the basis of 8,000 practicing veterinarians, there is thus, in round numbers, only 1 veterinarian to every 625 livestock owners, and to every 25,000 animals. Nor do these comparisons include the veterinary needs of the extensive poultry industry or of thousands of pet animals, notably dogs and cats, for which hundreds of well-equipped veterinary hospitals are maintained.

Diffusion of Knowledge: A Basic Public Policy

From the foregoing data it is clear that the services of research workers and practicing veterinarians must be greatly extended if current knowledge concerning livestock health is to be most beneficially applied. Moreover, the knowledge is constantly increasing. In dealing with this condition, the Bureau of Animal Industry and other agencies of the United States Department of Agriculture have long fostered the policy of sponsoring not only veterinary education and research, but also the distribution of useful knowledge in those fields to all interested persons.

To obtain wide and prompt diffusion of information, the Bureau utilizes at least 10 main channels, comprising publications, extension agencies, motion pictures, lantern slides, film strips, posters, exhibits, public demonstrations and addresses, and radio broadcasts. Veterinarians and other specialists of the Bureau have prepared approximately 100 publications dealing with animal diseases and parasites, including those of poultry. Periodic revision keeps the information up to date. Other Department agencies and State experiment stations, having similar information policies, likewise have issued numerous publications and other material.

In contrast to the specific personal services rendered by veterinarians, the information distributed through publications and other such means is usually of a more general character. It is intended chiefly to familiarize livestock owners and others with the characteristics of diseases, their dangers, the importance of prevention, and the value of sound, tested methods in dealing with them. It emphasizes the need and value of qualified veterinary services as compared with methods that are wasteful, ineffective, and sometimes cruel. One result of information services has been a greater familiarity on the part of the general public–consumers as well as producers–with animal diseases transmissible to human beings. Rabies, tuberculosis, anthrax, and trichinosis are typical examples of such diseases. Constructive legislation for the protection of both man and animals has resulted from this greater knowledge.

Types of Informational Material

In general, the most convenient sources of information on veterinary and livestock subjects are Federal and State publications. Most of them are supplied on request, either free or at nominal cost. They may also be consulted in libraries, in the offices of county agents, and in veterinary institutions. Publications on animal diseases or related subjects are of three general types: (1) So-called popular publications intended for laymen, (2) technical papers intended for veterinarians and research workers, and (3) official reports and similar publications dealing with such matters as the status of animal diseases, the progress of eradication work, and losses caused by disease; this last type of publication is commonly distributed only to public officials and practicing veterinarians, but it is available also to other interested persons.

Exhibits, lantern slides, film strips, and posters acquaint the public with pertinent facts concerning animal diseases and veterinary services. Pictorial presentation is especially suitable for showing typical symptoms of diseases. A collection of 12 veterinary posters, known as the Livestock Health Series, issued by the Bureau of Animal Industry, has met with favour among both professional workers and livestock owners.

On frequent occasions veterinarians and officials engaged in extension work have cooperated in arranging for demonstrations to familiarize livestock owners with the characteristics of diseases in combating which community cooperation is desirable. Commonly the extension worker arranges for the meeting and explains the purpose and value of the service to be rendered. The veterinarian then conducts the demonstration and supplies technical information.

In conducting tick-eradication work in the South, much of the preliminary information was conveyed by motion pictures shown by means of a portable projector (Fig. 1). Pictures shown in this way proved to be highly effective also in combating tuberculosis, hog cholera, and several other diseases. A widely distributed talking motion picture, Livestock and Mankind, produced by the Department of Agriculture, is essentially an illustrated lecture by John R. Mohler, Chief of the Bureau of Animal Industry. It deals in large measure with the development and uses of scientific knowledge concerning livestock. Motion pictures commonly serve two useful purposes– they help to draw a crowd as well as furnishing information in an interesting and often dramatic manner.

In recent years radio has been a useful informational ally of veterinary science. The speed of radio transmission makes it especially valuable when dealing with outbreaks of dangerous animal maladies. The radio was used successfully in warning livestock owners of the presence of foot-and-mouth disease in the United States during the outbreaks of 1924, 1925, and 1929. In dealing with such a highly infectious malady, a saving of even an hour's time is important. A broadcast notification may prevent the marketing of diseased animals or their distribution on large range pastures where they could expose other animals to infection.

In the radio field, the Farm Credit Administration has distributed four transcriptions of talks on veterinary subjects presented in human-interest style. Prepared on disk records, the talks, averaging

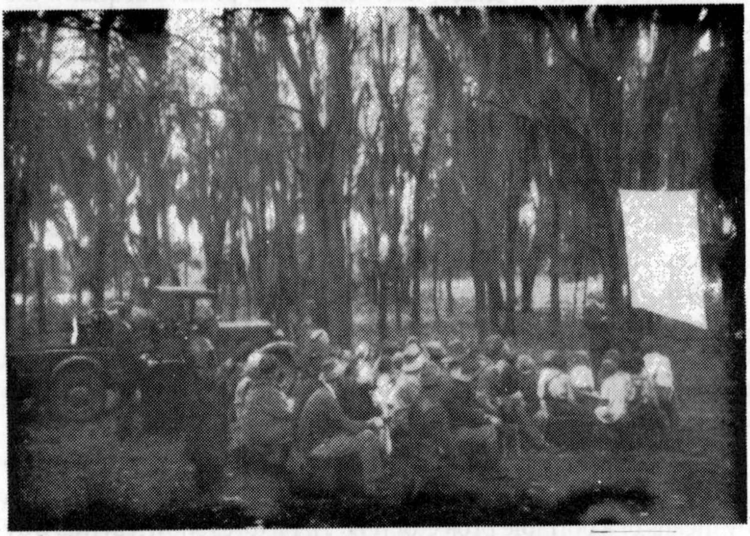

Fig. 1: Preparing to show a motion picture on cattle-tick eradication, projected by portable equipment. This method has proved to be highly effective in furthering public understanding of Department disease-eradication projects and obtaining the necessary cooperation.

about 15 minutes each, deal with hog cholera, cattle ticks, foot-and-mouth disease, and Federal meat inspection. Several hundred radio stations have either already used the transcriptions or applied for them. In recent years also, officers in charge of arrangements at meetings of veterinary medical associations have arranged for the broadcasting of important addresses.

Another type of information concerning animal diseases is contained in a series of handbooks relating to agriculture sponsored by Federal and State officials. These publications contain the names and addresses of officials and agencies prepared to render services along various lines; many States, for example, maintain laboratories where specimens of diseased tissues and small animals may be examined as a basis for diagnosis and remedial measures. As an aid in acquainting livestock owners with effective dips and disinfectants, the Bureau of Animal Industry issues lists of such products as have been approved for official use, giving the names of the various commercial brands and specifying the diseases or parasites against which each product is effective.

As a guide to persons contemplating buying or selling transactions that will involve interstate shipments of livestock, the Bureau of Animal Industry has prepared a compilation entitled "State Sanitary Requirements Governing the Admission of Livestock." This publication, printed in convenient handbook form, contains digests of State laws on this subject and gives the requirements of each State with respect to necessary certificates, tests, inspections, and dippings applicable to various species of domestic animals, including dogs and poultry.

Diseases common to horses and cattle are discussed also in two Congressional documents entitled "Diseases of the Horse" and "Diseases of Cattle," which may be obtained from United States Senators and Representatives who have quotas of the books for distribution or by purchase from the Superintendent of Documents, Government Printing Office, Washington, D.C.

As a part of the cooperative Federal-State campaigns against bovine tuberculosis and brucellosis (Bang's disease), inspectors who make tests for these diseases furnish considerable information to livestock owners, both verbally and through printed matter left with them. Combating brucellosis necessitates a number of sanitary precautions to prevent reinfection, and the veterinary inspectors discuss the various requirements with each livestock owner and obtain from him a signed agreement indicating that the owner understands the procedures to be followed and will carry them out. In campaigns that involve the testing of thousands of herds, these personal contacts have far-reaching informational value.

To help bring about a broader knowledge of Federal meat inspection, the Bureau of Animal Industry, which conducts this service, has provided its inspectors with educational literature, including the text for a 10-minute talk on the subject. The same material is available to lecturers and other persons in need of authoritative information on safeguards to the meat food supply.

Large Expenditures for Ineffective Remedies

A further service that science seeks to render is that of cautioning the public against expenditures for drugs and nostrums that are worthless in preventing or treating animal maladies. Although most manufacturers distribute dependable goods and advertise their merits truthfully, others have been found by the Food and Drug Administration of the Federal Security Agency to make exaggerated claims wholly unwarranted in the light of scientific knowledge and tests. Some of the advertising has led worried stock owners to believe that the so-called remedies would cure diseases for which there is no known cure.

Estimates of the money spent in the United States for ineffective proprietary remedies for animal diseases indicate that the amount still exceeds 10 million dollars a year. This huge expenditure is largely wasted. The spending of half or even a smaller fraction of the amount for veterinary services would be vastly more productive in accomplishing the desired results. It is highly important also to distinguish clearly between the purpose for which different biological products and chemicals are intended. Some are diagnostic, their sole value being to detect disease conditions; other have immunizing value; and still others, although not many, have curative properties. In the treatment of internal parasites, products known as anthelmintics, when properly used, are beneficial in eliminating all or most of the parasites from affected animals, but periodic use may be necessary to prevent further infestation.

Accurate diagnosis of a disease or ailment should always precede any attempt at treatment, both in order that the treatment may be intelligently applied and to save the expense of administering ineffective or needless remedies. Recently a Federal veterinarian investigated promiscuous dosing of sheep, allegedly for worm parasites, in an area in the Southwest. Inspection of the animals together with several post mortem examinations showed that the parasites for which treatment was being given did not exist in that area. The incident illustrates how time, money, and labour may be needlessly expended.

Practical Value of Animal-Disease Information

Persons about to engage in raising livestock or those who have recently undertaken it should inform themselves as promptly as possible concerning diseases, parasites, and other ailments likely to affect the species of animal concerned. This is desirable both to safeguard the stock owner's individual investment and as a protection for all livestock in the community.

Conservative estimates indicate that animal diseases and parasites cost the average livestock owner about $40 a year, partly through the death of animals (Fig. 2) but even more through impaired efficiency (Fig. 3), slower growth, and reduced market value. Animals that are seriously affected with disease at some time in their lives generally cost more to raise and bring less money when sold than consistently healthy stock.

The most successful livestock owners appear to have prospered in large measure because they have built up effective barriers against disease, utilized veterinary services, and otherwise sought to reduce losses from the inroads of diseases and pests. The stockmen who have paid the heaviest toll in disease losses are usually those least able to sustain such losses.

It is especially desirable that livestock owners should be informed regarding diseases that spread rapidly and are likely to endanger animals on neighboring premises. For example, any

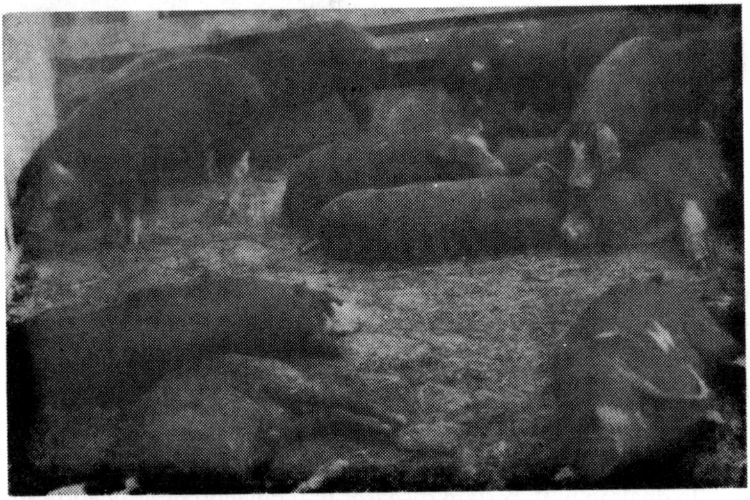

Fig. 2: Disease takes its toll. Typical appearance of a herd of swine when hog cholera strikes. Too late now for treatment; the loss will be several hundred dollars.

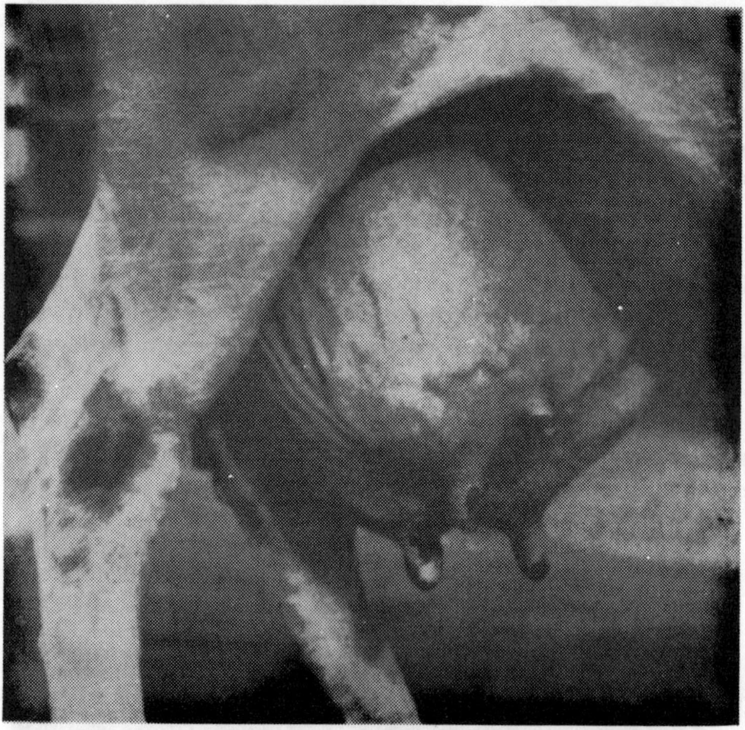

Fig. 3: A case of chronic mastitis. Only about half of this udder is functioning. Dead animals by no means represent all the losses caused by disease.

condition suspected of being foot-and-mouth disease should be reported immediately, by telephone or telegraph, to the nearest veterinarian (Fig. 4). Success in keeping this disease out of the country or immediately stamping out its invasions means large savings to the livestock industry. Stockmen are therefore urged to familiarize themselves with the characteristics of this and other serious maladies.

In dealing with certain diseases that develop rapidly and can be prevented by immunization, such as hog cholera, prompt action is essential. When outbreaks have appeared on neighboring farms prompt application of the preventive serum treatment may be the

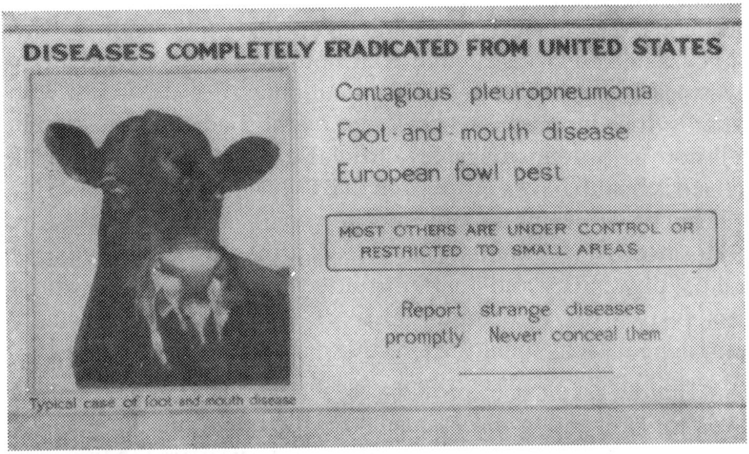

Fig. 4: An exhibit panel designed to acquaint livestock owners with the symptoms of foot-and-mouth disease so that they may recognize and report this foreign malady promptly should it appear in the United States.

means of saving large numbers of animals not previously immunized.

The practice of leaving dead animals unburied is especially dangerous for the reason that dogs or birds may feed on the carcasses and carry the infection far and wide. When animals are crowded together, the chances for diseases and parasites to spread are increased.

Benefits of Broad Public Understanding

It has been shown that livestock owners in the United States have readily available (1) extensive factual material that acquaints them with the principal disease problems and methods of prevention and control, and (2) the personal services of veterinarians engaged in private practice or representing local, State, or Federal agencies.

The Bureau of Animal Industry does not concur in the belief occasionally expressed that information on animal diseases should be distributed only or primarily to veterinarians and applied by them in response to calls for their services. As a public agency, the

Bureau is prepared to furnish information to all interested persons so that the largest possible number will be adequately informed concerning the problems underlying animal health, for these problems have a bearing on public safety and public welfare. This policy is deemed constructive from a public standpoint and fair to livestock owners and veterinary practitioners. It is also in line with what is done by public agencies and by the medical profession in relation to human diseases. Official publications concerning livestock health have emphasized that the diagnosis of disease, the treatment of animals, and any necessary surgery should be performed by veterinarians who have a thorough knowledge of animal physiology and are trained to render such services. Under this system the informational work and veterinary services supplement each other in an effective manner.

The net result is to provide, on the one hand, a dependable basis for preventing diseases and, on the other, the professional selection and use of proper procedures for combating them when they occur. Under the policies outlined, the production of domestic animals in the United States, already a sound enterprise, is proceeding with increasing safety.

INDEX